PRAIS

Marijuana
A LOVE STORY

"As a grandmother in the movement, I am increasingly concerned that the space for small farmers and businesses is shrinking in the face of big corporations and corporate profits. Jensen's and Silvaggio's book explains what is happening in the cannabis space, why it is important to protect legacy producers, and what we need to do to keep the dream alive. A must read." **—MADELINE MARTINEZ, NORML Board of Directors; NORML Women's Alliance Chair; Executive Director, Oregon NORML; owner-founder of the World Famous Cannabis Café**

"*Marijuana: A Love Story* reminds us of what first motivated our calls for cannabis legalization—awe and love of the plant itself and the honest desire to use marijuana without being arrested." **—CONSTANCE BUMGARNER GEE, author of *Higher Education: Marijuana at the Mansion***

"*Marijuana: A Love Story* is many things: a unique book about a unique plant, a clear analysis of what has gone wrong with legalization and how to fix it, a wild look at the quirky culture that has grown up around it, and a love song not only to this plant but to all of evolution." **—LIERRE KEITH, author of *The Vegetarian Myth* and *Bright Green Lies***

"*Marijuana: A Love Story* reads like your best marijuana trip: funny, friendly, relaxing. Stories, jokes, and deep thoughts rise up then recede, intertwine and coalesce into a coherent experience. After reading this book, you'll feel, like Jimi Hendrix sang, not necessarily stoned, but beautiful." **— C. O. GREENE, a Humboldt County grower who must remain anonymous, because she's still growing, still underground, still resisting government and corporate control of her beloved plant**

Marijuana

A LOVE STORY

Derrick Jensen

AND

Tony Silvaggio

Red Elixir
Rhinebeck, New York

Paperback ISBN: 978-1-954744-55-4
eBook ISBN: 978-1-954744-56-1

Library of Congress Control Number: 2022932870

Book and cover design by Colin Rolfe

Red Elixir is an imprint of Monkfish Book Publishing Company

Red Elixir
22 East Market Street, Suite 304
Rhinebeck, NY 12572
(85) 876-4861
monkfishpublishing.com

Contents

CHAPTER 1

The Meeting

I'm riding shotgun. Tim drives. I glance into the right-side wing mirror, see a cop coming up behind us.

I sit up stiff in my seat, stare straight ahead, think, "This is what an innocent passenger looks like, right?" Then I realize how ridiculous that is. On an interstate you relax, hang out, pass the time. So I pick up the paperback I was reading a while ago and pretend to read. Isn't that what you do in a car if you're not breaking any laws?

Tim hasn't noticed my actions. I don't think he's even noticed the cop. I see him glance in the rearview mirror, then back to the front.

Nothing. He doesn't even stop speeding.

He must have read my mind. He says, "I'm only going seventy-four."

I don't understand what he's saying. I don't understand why I agreed to ride with him. I don't even understand why we're in this particular vehicle. It's a black, decades-old Suburban, converted to run on bio-diesel, with anti-imperial bumper stickers plastered all over the back. U.S. OUT OF NORTH AMERICA. END CORPORATE RULE. SURE, YOU CAN TRUST THE GOVERNMENT—ASK AN INDIAN. At least he doesn't have any stickers about marijuana.

We should have brought my mom's car. It's a Prius, for God's sake. Why would a cop stop a Prius? And we should have brought my mom along. She could ride shotgun and I'd sit in the back. Nobody's going to stop a Prius with a seventy-year-old woman in the passenger seat.

I pretend to read my book. But I keep looking off the page to the right, to the mirror. The cop is getting close.

Tim almost laughs, then gives me a friendly side-eye and slightly shakes his head.

I don't want to be that clichéd character from every disaster movie who starts to whine as soon as things get tough. So I don't tell Tim to slow down. I don't tell him to keep his hands at ten and two.

I don't freak out.

At least on the outside.

I glance again at the mirror.

The cop is gone.

I look to my left. The cop is passing us. Tim looks over at him, smiling ingenuously.

The cop doesn't even look our way.

Tim parks at a farm house. We get out, walk to the back of the Suburban. Tim pops it open, reaches in to grab two black carry-on duffel bags. He hands one to me. I almost laugh out loud. Another movie cliché. Anyone who has ever seen an action movie knows that when you see two men arrive at a lonely farmhouse in a black Suburban and carry black carry-on duffel bags to the door, the bags contain either money or drugs.

But never transport both at the same time, Tim tells me. Never transport both at the same time.

Mario greets us at the door, invites us in. I look around. I'm not sure what I thought a house would look like where a drug transaction was going to take place, but this wasn't it. This looks exactly like what it is: the house of a small farmer.

Mario opens a coat closet and Tim puts the duffel bags inside.

Tim says, "Here's four pounds each of Trainwreck, Blueberry Kush, and Granddaddy Purple."

Mario leaves the room for a minute, comes back with a small courier bag—black, of course. He hands it to Tim, says, "Here's your money from last time. Belinda came down and got it, sent it East. It's thirty-five K. You got two K instead of three on one of the pounds, since the buds were a bit small."

"Fucking yuppies," Tim says.

I look back and forth between them.

Mario says, "Everybody loves trophy buds, since they look cool, but it's kind of ridiculous. The smoke is the same on small buds, and you grind 'em all before you smoke anyway. And big buds have a lot more lumber."

"Lumber?" I say.

Tim says, "Stem in the middle. Wasted, really. So in fact they're getting less smoke for their money." He gives me a look that says, "People, what are you going to do about them?"

There's a slight pause before Tim says, "Would you like to see Mario's grow?"

When Mario opens the door to his grow—it's in a special room built inside his barn—I don't so much smell the marijuana as find myself enveloped in a blanket of sharp, sweet, earthy, skunky funk with overtones ranging from freshly-bruised pine to grapefruit, to the faintest hints of cat piss and baby shit. I've never smelled anything like it. Apart from the marijuana scent I remember from other people's smoke at concerts when I was a teen-ager—I never smoked, myself—I had no idea what to expect. But I like this smell. I like it a lot. Except for the cat piss and baby shit.

The room is roughly ten by twenty and lit by several big fixtures hanging from the ceiling. The walls are painted bright white, presumably for maximum reflectivity. There are only six plants, each in a thirty-gallon, gray, plastic tote filled with potting soil. The plants are huge, with multiple woody stems leading to branches reaching up to a thick canopy of deep green leaves and long masses of flowers—Mario tells me you call these masses *colas*—all waving in the breeze—wind, really—from a series of fans attached to the upper corners of the room.

I love it all: the smell, the leaves blowing in the wind, the sturdy stems. Hell, let's call them what they are—trunks.

Mario looks at me, closely. I can tell he knows what I'm thinking. He says, "So, Tim tells me you want to learn how to grow."

*

That was fifteen years ago. Much has changed since then. Now, due to legalization, I could hold a one-pound bag of marijuana in one hand and a bag of doughnuts in the other, walk into the sheriff's office, hand them the latter and walk out with the former. Later, I could report to the sheriff that someone broke into my house and stole my pot. I have in fact done exactly that.

Not long ago the walls of grow shops were lined with posters of tomatoes and other fruits and vegetables alongside signs reading, "If you discuss anything illegal, you'll be asked to leave." This invariably led to strange conversations about what fertilizers customers should buy to make their tomato flowers grow bigger and stronger-smelling and have—uh, you know, more, uh—tomato effects.

Back then there were rumors about grow shops, how they were really fronts for the Drug Enforcement Agency, and if you paid by check or credit card the cops would go to your address and bust your ass. Of course, all the sensible growers knew this was crap. The *real* way the DEA was going to get you was by surveillance cameras outside the store—see them up there?—recording your license number and using that to find your address. And, well, you know the rest. But the really serious growers knew even this was crap. Instead, the DEA inserted RFID chips into the packaging of every item, from every bag of Happy Frog potting soil to every gallon of Tiger Bloom fertilizer. These chips then relayed information to a GPS system that would track whatever you bought to wherever your grow room was, after which the cops would come—and, again, you know the rest.

Nobody ever claimed pot doesn't make you paranoid.

Nowadays you can openly buy more or less every marijuana accessory in industrial quantities on the internet.

The biggest change, from the perspective of those within marijuana culture, is that nobody, not even master growers like Tim or Mario, get $3,000/lb. wholesale anymore. The best growers get $2,000/lb., and the price is falling fast. Many, like Tim, Mario, and Belinda have been forced to quit. Tim now substitute-teaches, Mario works construction, which is hard on his old bones, and Belinda works the night shift changing bed pans in a hospice.

Marijuana legalization—that long-deferred dream of stoners everywhere—is conquering the nation. Recreational use is now legal in nineteen states plus the District of Columbia. Marijuana has been decriminalized in another thirteen states plus the US Virgin Islands. Most other states have legalized the plant for medicinal use, with only four states maintaining complete prohibition.

This is all great, right? No longer will people be imprisoned for decades for possession of a plant. No longer will people be denied marijuana needed for medical treatment. Heck, people who just want to get high will have easy, safe access.

Unfortunately, especially because of how it's being done, legalization comes at a cost. In this case it probably means the end of the "marijuana culture" that has evolved in the Emerald Triangle of California—Humboldt, Trinity, and Mendocino counties—a culture known for growing the best marijuana in the world, a culture that is, for now, as storied and wild and often just plain crazy as the cowboy culture of the Old West (and that has existed longer than did the golden era of cowboys). It's a culture disappearing before our eyes.

It also means the corporate takeover of the industry, from growth to distribution to sales.

As Mario said to me, "I've dreamt of legalization since I started growing in the 1970s. But now, the way it's happening, I wish I'd never pushed for it."

He's not alone.

It's not merely marijuana culture in California at risk. Recently someone from Kansas, who has spent most of his adult life trying to make a living as an independent mycologist, told me that until Colorado legalized, growing marijuana had paid his rent. Never until that moment had I considered how difficult it would be to make a living as an independent mycologist. In Kansas.

*

Last night I was at my mom's. She's eighty-five now, not seventy, and she has indeed accompanied me on a couple of pot runs, but more for the chance to go on a beautiful drive than to act as a human shield. We were watching television, and I was, of course, flipping through the channels. I came across Bill Maher talking about marijuana with Vicente Fox, former president of Mexico.

Maher said, "In this state we just legalized it. And I happen to know a grower. . . . He told me the price dropped, like overnight, from $1,600/lb. to $200." The audience applauded. Maher continued, "So there was some good news, ladies and gentlemen, this horrible week."

Fox responded, "You move that massive amount of money from criminals into government through paying taxes. This is the difference: sitting on your side with [El] Chapo Guzman or sitting here with farmers and businessmen that are today running that new industry. This is the paradigm that we want to change in Mexico."[1]

This exchange well encapsulates current mainstream thinking on legalization and encapsulates as well the understanding that legalization is not, as many legalization advocates would like to believe, primarily about "freeing the sacred herb" but rather is primarily motivated by government attempts to capture a revenue stream.

The question becomes, from whom is this revenue stream being captured? Bill Maher gives one answer to this question, as the "grower" (a.k.a. small farmer) he mentions has seen his gross income drop by more than 87 percent "overnight." This actually means his gross income has dropped by 100 percent, since he can no longer keep farming.

Bill Maher calls this "good news." I'm not sure the farmer would agree.

I do suppose there is some good news, however, in that the farmer has learned a new phrase: "Would you like fries with that?"

---

[1] Fox became an editor at the marijuana magazine *High Times* around the time the organization lost its soul, started doing things like defunding marijuana music, including even *Reggae on the River* here in the heart of the Emerald Triangle.

It should not surprise us that Fox, a politician, was being disingenuous, since disingenuous is the default state for politicians. Fox talked about "farmers and businessmen" "running the new industry." But Bill Maher had just made it clear that honest-to-goodness farmers are being driven out of "the new [sic] industry." The winners in this transfer of wealth are the usually white, usually-already-wealthy-businesspeople who are taking advantage of this new Green Rush. Colorado's legal industry is already controlled by only a handful of wealthy economic entities. Same with Oregon. And is anyone surprised that the sugar-and-pineapple-baron Baldwin Brothers who essentially own Maui were given rare permits to grow on the island, granting them a central role in the new *legal* cartel controlling marijuana there?

Fox equates "criminals" with El Chapo Guzman, former leader of the Sinaloa Cartel, known for sending nearly 200 tons of cocaine to the United States, as well as equally unimaginable amounts of methamphetamines, heroin, fentanyl, marijuana, and so on. The Cartel is also known for beheading those who get in their way and filming themselves dissolving their victims' bodies in lye, then posting this on the internet as a warning to others.

Scary stuff, obviously, and clearly atrocities. Transfers of wealth away from those who commit atrocities are good things.

But the criminals I know are a little different. Recall Tim, Mario, Belinda, the independent mycologist. And there are so many others.

Six or seven years ago I spoke with Moira, over a big pile of waffle-cut fries. I asked how she got started.

She said, "I was a single mom with four kids. I had a good job but had to quit to take care of my mom during her last three months. The company had promised to hire me back, but by the time my mom died they'd found someone else." She stopped, dipped a fry into a blob of ketchup, looked at it for a few moments, then said, "Best thing that ever happened to me." She popped the fry in her mouth, chewed, swallowed. She continued, "Before, I was barely able to get by and the kids were home alone too many hours, but now I support us pretty well. And I love what I do. In taking care of my mom I learned the value of comfort, and here was a plant that provided comfort in so many ways.

There is great comfort in being able to buy school pictures without looking for pennies under the couch and feeling heartbroken when there aren't enough of them.

"I've been able to help other single moms, too, just as other women helped me get started. I have a small scene, only four lights. Some people run bigger scenes but it's all we need. We help each other.

"I love watching the plants grow their proud green leaves. I love starting the clones, the babies. I have so much respect for the life in the soil as it nurtures the plant. But my favorite part is the trimming. A few of my friends come over; I imagine it might be like quilting bees. We sit in silence sometimes, we talk sometimes. We share and we create a finished product of quality and value.

"I do think that having something to offer of value has helped me feel more of my own personal value. When you work so hard for poor wages you feel unwhole, like you are not a person worth anything. Like you are a failure before you even start.

"The plant has made me whole in that regard. Did you know that 'to heal' means 'to make whole'? The plant has healed me."

Then there's the grower I just spoke to who told me, "I grow cannabis because I love plants, all plants. I grew up in a perfect microcosm of the abusive culture we find ourselves in today. The garden and wilderness were always my refuge. Therefore, I found the perfect craft with the cannabis plant to provide a means to support myself. I've always felt incredibly lucky to be able to grow a plant that is fairly easy to grow and worth so much money. But I don't do this for money. I grow cannabis because the plant and its worth allow me to make a living through a relationship with a plant. The monetary value of the plant allowed me to have a very small cultivation. The small farm fostered the ability to form a close relationship with the plant. If I had a large farm, the intimacy wouldn't be there. Each strain has a personality. They can be serious, funny, friendly, poetic, sassy, angry, or bossy! Sitting in the garden in the cool mornings with my plants, listening to them, has given me such peace and precious memories. I always hire gentle and kind people—mostly women—to work for me, and I pay them well. When we work in the field together, we laugh and tell funny stories while we deleaf, prune, or trellis. When we work with the plants outside, I often feel what I would describe as an ancient sense of peace, a feeling that I imagine our pre-civilization ancestors felt while gathering plants. The economic value of cannabis in today's world commands a respect that I imagine ancient peoples who didn't participate in capitalism had for all plants. I'm grateful to have lived a life having a deep relationship with a plant. I actually don't consume cannabis much, but I love her deeply."

I spoke with another woman who said, "I've known so many women who've grown cannabis to try to escape from violent relationships—violent men—and to be able to stay home and raise their children right. Unfortunately, a lot of these women haven't lasted, because we've found in marijuana culture many of the same attitudes we see in the culture at large. But we exist, and persist. Pre-legalization we were more prevalent, small-scale medical cultivators who sang to our plants, giggled with our children, grew our own food. There are still a few of us, but I fear for our future."

Or there's the criminal Jessica, an impoverished painter ("Is there any other kind?" she asks) who never thought much about marijuana until a friend in Hartford, Connecticut, said, "You live in Arcata, California? You're sitting on a gold mine." Soon she—like so many other people in this region—was mailing bud across the country and around the world. As a consequence, she was able to pay for necessary medical and dental procedures, something she'd never before been able to do. "The first time I took a box of bud into the post office," she told me, "I was so scared I was shaking. I even wore loose-fitting clothes in the hope my shaking wouldn't be quite so noticeable. The clerk still noticed the shaking, and said, 'It's cold out there today, isn't it?'"

I'm not suggesting that every person involved in the marijuana trade is a criminal of the genus *Cuddly*. There are shits in marijuana culture like there are shits in every culture. Theft is a big problem. Many outdoor growers sleep in their grows from August to harvest, guns at the ready. I know a woman who walked outside and saw thieves taking her pot. She started screaming. One of the thieves ran up to her and pistol whipped her. Fortunately, her roommate emerged from their pit outhouse, pants just-pulled-up-but-not-fastened, and fired his shotgun into the air. And yes, this means he carried his shotgun with him even to the john. I know another woman who made a deal with a land-owner where she'd do all the work on his grow, and they'd split the money 25 percent for her, 75 percent for him. (Side-note on the sexism in marijuana culture: the standard for this sort of arrangement is that if the worker is a woman, she gets 25 percent—and if a man, he gets 30 percent.) But in this case, she got 0 percent. When he got the money for the harvest, he didn't give her a dime. And there was nothing she could do. Other women are, of course, like everywhere else in this culture, sexually abused.

There can be profound specialization among thieves. There are those who make a living scouting outdoor grows and rating the secu-rity, then not stealing marijuana themselves but rather selling maps to other thieves.

And we've all heard of marijuana growers arrested holding two kilos of coke, $100,000 in cash, and several AR-15s, all behind barbed wire patrolled by trained attack dogs. They really do exist.

There also exist those who grow simply to feed their addictions, whether these addictions are to meth, heroin, cocaine, prescription pills, computer games, or most likely, money or power. Of course, one also could ask whether many of the winners in the new legalized green rush are feeding their own addictions to money and/or power. I'm sure the Baldwin Brothers, with their sugar/pineapple/real estate holdings, are not searching under couches for pennies.

But for every criminal of the genus *Nasty-ass motherfucker*, there are plenty of single mothers, independent mycologists, painters, sculptors, home health care providers, environmentalists, and those who have simply fallen in love with the plant.

And their way of life is being destroyed.

Part of the sorrow of this is that the destruction of marijuana cul-ture—and the looming incapacity of these people to make a living—is not entirely pre-ordained. Fairly straightforward fixes could be put in place to allow small operators to continue.

For example, as California was devising its regulations for legalization, strong arguments and counterarguments were put forward as to whether the upper limit on the size of outdoor grows should be one acre or ten acres. Either of these limits would have prevented huge corporations from putting in megafarms in the Central Valley where, instead of seeing mile after mile of rice and soybeans and almonds, you'll see mile after mile of monocropped marijuana.

But at the last moment, the government of California did what governments so often do and surprised the naïve by removing limits altogether.

Good-bye mom and pop. Hello transnational corporations.

I spoke with a long-time grower who said, "Smaller governing entities like city councils and county boards of supervisors are also responsible for devastating small farmers, changing licensing requirements monthly to exhaust all funds of the small guys. This happened to me. I lost so much hard-earned money trying to follow the law that I eventually exhausted everything I'd saved from running a very successful cannabis company and had to take a trimming job. It was humiliating. The League of Cities in California planned this scenario in detail years before 'legalization.' Even medium grows in my town are taxed, regulated, and licensed out of business. Our county is charging back taxes on pre-legalization compassion programs for cannabis donated to people, many of whom are veterans in need. These taxes are just one thing crippling legal cannabis companies now. I could go on and on. It so often feels like this is some sort of punishment for all these underground growers getting away with being not under their control for all of those years."

Or maybe they just want to make sure the money goes to the already wealthy.

One of the problems is that economies of scale—where the larger your operation, the lower your unit costs—make it almost impossible for artisans, and community, and living wages to continue in the face of mass production. For decades marijuana culture and the craft of

11

growing fine marijuana were protected from this logic *by the law*: marijuana's illegality prevented concentration of ownership and production because those with deep pockets couldn't build acre after acre of greenhouses or grow outdoor fields rivaling corn, wheat, or soybeans. They—or at least their laborers—would be arrested.

But while illegality could not destroy marijuana culture, legalization is. Just today I heard a grower mirror what Bill Maher's grower said, "I used to get $3,000/lb. for my pot, and now it's $800. I need at least $1,000 to break even."

Wages for workers, traditionally fairly high, are dropping. Also today, I spoke with a trimmer who used to make $250 per pound of trimmed bud, and now makes $100. That's still better than what trimmers get in corporate trim factories, which pay migrant workers $50/lb. And underground trimmers often get to do their work at home, which makes it an ideal job for single mothers, who can take care of their children while they work or work while their children sleep or do homework, and who can drop the trimming in a heartbeat when one toddler suddenly goes silent in the kitchen, which of course means one child is eating the dog's food while, simultaneously, the other decides the kitty litter is really a sandbox. Regulations under legalization prohibit trimmers from taking home the pot, thus making mothers leave home, forcing them to pay for babysitters.

Legalization is poised to devastate local communities. Prior to legalization, one out of every five houses in Arcata, California, was a grow scene. Businesspeople from dentists to veterinarians to car dealers didn't—and don't—blink when handed thousands of dollars in cash for services rendered. (Not only do they not blink, but many offer cash discounts. One grower told me that when she paid her rather large power bill all in ten-dollar bills, the clerk laughed and said, "I see you've been selling lots of dime bags.") Marijuana essentially *is* the economy of several counties. Without marijuana, these economies will collapse. Indeed, with legalization, many have. It surprised no one in my tiny town that several restaurants closed in the months after legalization. Not only do people in this community have less disposable income, but I'd wager at least some of these restaurants had existed to launder marijuana money.

A grower told me, "Practically every cool small business in Santa Cruz was funded with cannabis dollars, and back in the day, cannabis dollars built pretty much everything in Big Sur. With the crash of the cannabis economy that's not going to continue."

The bigger problem is that what we're seeing in northern California—and Kansas, and elsewhere—is a modern retelling of the takeover of organic farming by Big Ag with the USDA release of federally approved organic standards in the 1990s, where small, traditionally organic farms were priced out of becoming certified through an expensive process big corporations could easily afford but family farmers could not. And it's a retelling of, more broadly, the destruction of family farms by Big Ag from the 1950s on. It's the story of independent booksellers driven out of business by conglomerates that are in turn eventually driven out of business by Amazon. Heck, it's the story of the Luddites, who rebelled against the takeover and destruction of their communal craft of weaving through the forced introduction of mechanical looms by big capitalists. It was no longer possible to make a living at that craft. If we go even further back, it's the story of the destruction of the guilds by the rise of capitalism.

It is the story of the concentration of wealth at the expense of craftspeople and communities.

The questions become: Have any of these cultures based on local geography and craft been able to withstand the intrusion of larger corporate interests? Has it happened even once? Is it possible?

Well, in the case of marijuana culture, there may be some fairly straightforward processes by which state and federal governments can indeed protect small growers and end the war on weed without it turning into a war on small family growers. This book will lay out some of these processes.

Whether or not these processes are put in place—and whether or not marijuana culture is able to continue—will depend on how much pressure American citizens put on those in power, and it will depend on whether we can force those in power to serve local communities rather than larger corporate interests.

So, I don't know. Is this book a call for action? Is it a description of historical processes? Is it an elegy for a wild and wacky culture being ground underfoot by big capital?

Perhaps it is all of these.

One final warning for now. Before any of you jump on the Bill Maher bandwagon that the collapse of the price of marijuana is a good thing, please consider that Fox didn't mention prices dropping. He mentioned a transfer of wealth. The money won't go to consumers. It will go to governments and to businesspeople. Just like the farmer gets a pittance for corn, with every entity on the distribution chain taking its *mordida*, so too the price at point of consumption will remain what it was, with all sorts of institutional and governmental entities wetting their beaks, and the farmer getting the financial equivalent of a wet willie. And even if marijuana's final price did drop, ask yourself how large-scale agriculture has served the quality of food you get. When was the last time you ate a strawberry? No, not an object that looked like a strawberry, didn't have much smell, and tasted like cardboard. A real strawberry. Or a peach. A real one, with a taste that ties you to a hot summer afternoon in your fourteenth year, sitting cross-legged in the shade of a tree with juice running down your chin and falling on your folded legs, and a smell that stays with you still. When was the last time you had a watermelon that tasted like a watermelon?

Until I moved to northern California, I always hated berries. Or rather I never cared about them. What's there to care about? Small tasteless sacks of watery juice in tiny overpriced baskets. But now I live in berry country. I pick them. I buy them from an organic blueberry farm a mile or so from my house. Like the bears I see almost every day here, I gorge on berries, till—and I'm sorry if this is too much information—my poop runs as dark blue as the bear poop I have to avoid in the forest, as dark blue as the bird poop I see splattered across the forest floor, as dark blue as the berries themselves.

Last summer I stopped at the local feed store to pick up some soil for my plants. On the way out I saw someone had erected a small table and was selling home-grown heirloom tomatoes. I bought some.

My feeling on tomatoes has always mirrored my feeling on berries. They're basically cardboard-tasting gut plugs, to be added as *pro forma* condiments to other meals. The attraction is primarily visual.

I bit into a tomato.

I suddenly wondered why anyone had ever bothered to invent candy. Why would you do so when you can eat something so profoundly delicious, so profoundly moving, as this? I suddenly understood those for whom cooking and eating are art forms. The flavors were powerful, subtle, shifting moment by moment, and I simultaneously wanted each moment not to end and for the next moment to come rushing toward me.

The same can be true for marijuana. Consider these descriptions written by a pot connoisseur for heirloom strains of marijuana grown by someone who loves the plants and who tends to them individually: "This strain reminds me why those who have been saying pot is a hallucinogen are correct. This is powerful, dreamy, and trippy. The trip is shiny, chrome-plated, and long lasting. It makes me remember how I felt when I first started getting high." Or "Crisp, understated, yet powerful. It's a good daily driver when I still need to function. Would be great for non-smokers." Or "It takes you way up and then brings you down a little washed out. I would recommend it for seasoned professionals who aren't bothered by seeing the occasional lizard person."

We all know what corporations have done to our food. Do we want the same done to our marijuana?

CHAPTER 2

The Mismatched Couple

For a time, I was the worst grower in the world. Not because my teachers weren't the best, for they were. Instead, the problem was a combination of my own congenital stubbornness, an almost-complete inability to learn except by repeatedly messing up, and an uncommon lack of common sense.

I overwatered, underwatered, overfed, underfed. If there was a way to mess things up, I did it. Several times. That's how I learn. Eventually. In the meantime, the plants were small, the buds tiny.

I thought I'd go to some online forums (back before Facebook destroyed them) and compare my bud size to those of others.

This was a mistake. Everyone else's buds were huge, their yields unbelievable. "My popcorn buds are the size of apricots and the top colas are as big as baseball bats. I get a pound and a half per plant indoors, and ten times that on my outdoor scene."

The more I read, the smaller my penis—I mean, buds—seemed.

There are a few reasons, however, that none of this bothered me as much as it could have.

The first is that I soon realized that lying about bud size and especially plant yield is rivaled only by lying about penis size. No, that isn't true; lying about yields is more extreme. It's as though men were claiming their penises were six feet tall and weighed 200 pounds (which would mean some men are complete dicks). Three-quarters of an ounce becomes four ounces, four ounces becomes a pound and a half. The size of a pencil becomes the size of a coke bottle, and a coke bottle becomes the size of a small tree.

The second is that by visiting these forums I discovered I was not in fact the worst grower in the world. For example, one guy posted a picture of a tiny, dead plant, with the comment: "What am I doing wrong? I water this plant four times a day and it's still dying." And several people posted pictures of beautiful huge male plants—complete with their little dingleberry blossoms—with the question, "Where are the buds?"

It's fine that a lot of people don't know that buds grow only on female plants. It's even fine that some inexperienced growers didn't know that. It just made them worse growers than I was.

So I felt better about that.

I still, however, had to ask myself the fundamental question: If even stoners—well, some stoners—can grow great buds, why can't I? How bad a grower do I have to be to not be able to grow a plant called *weed*? What's next, I fail at growing dandelions?

The third reason my comparative failure didn't bother me so much is that I was growing to neither get high nor get rich but rather to try to heal.

I'm pretty much a poster child for what Prop 215—legalizing marijuana for medicinal purposes in California—was supposed to be about. I've never in my life used an illegal drug. Same with alcohol. For crying out loud, I don't even drink caffeine except to stay awake when driving long distances. But I have Crohn's disease, one of the first half-dozen conditions that marijuana was found to help.

My first experience with marijuana was terrible. I was at a friend's house, and in great pain. I asked if she had anything for it. She handed me a marijuana cookie. I'd heard marijuana was good for pain, so I took it. She didn't tell me how strong it was. This next won't mean much to those who have never ingested a marijuana cookie and will mean quite a lot to those who have. She gave me an entire cookie.

I didn't notice anything for about an hour. I was driving—yes, she gave an entire marijuana cookie to someone who had never before ingested any mind-altering substance and then put him behind the wheel of a pickup truck—when the effects suddenly hit me.

I began to dream with my eyes open. Someone else was driving the truck while I watched. I watched other vehicles pass in the other direction. I watched the forest slide by. I watched my hands on the steering wheel. I participated in none of this. Finally, I heard my voice say, "I can't drive anymore," and I saw my hands turn the wheel slightly to the right and pull the truck to a stop. I saw a hand pull the door handle and saw the door open. Feet appeared and reached for the ground. I stood and started to walk. Or rather my field of vision rotated down toward the ground, and I saw first one shoed foot after another come into that field, as I saw myself move forward.

I spent the afternoon hallucinating. I don't remember most of what I saw. I mainly remember what I felt, which was terror. My main fear was that I would never come back. I remember hearing my voice say, perhaps every two or three minutes, "How much longer will this last?"

I remember thinking that if this lasted more than two or three days, I would kill myself. I remember wondering whether the books I had written were real, or if I had only dreamt I was a writer.

I hallucinated through the afternoon and into the evening. Finally that night, I was lucid enough to drive home. I went to bed. The next day I no longer hallucinated but found myself unable to think clearly. Even simple cognitive tasks required great effort, and more complex cognitive tasks were impossible. I remained stupid all through that next day and into the night: I suddenly understood how someone can vote for Republicans, or Democrats.

The day after, I could think again. I was back and immeasurably glad to be so.

That night, I suddenly realized I had been in absolutely no pain for the previous two and a half days.

That was when I became a believer in medical marijuana.

Tim came to visit. He looked at my buds. He said, "I've seen smaller."

I said, "Thank you, I guess."

He asked about my regimen. I told him. He made suggestions. Then he said, "But I don't think this is *entirely* your fault."

I said, "Thank you, I guess."

"Where'd you get your genetics?"

"My seeds?"

"Seeds, clones, whatever."

I told Tim how I'd gotten each strain. The stories fell into two categories: I bought the seeds from Europe, with the seeds sent hidden in a package of hard candy, or "I got them from some guy."

I just violated a fundamental rule of pot transportation: never reveal anyone's "stealth" means for packaging and mailing. But since the European website gives the option of overpaying for a small box of sweets under the category of "super-duper stealth," I don't think my comment is news to customs agents.

Tim listened patiently, then tilted his head toward his Suburban. We walked to the back, and he opened the hatch. Inside was a cooler, not surprisingly covered with bumper stickers: a photo of Geronimo with the caption, HOMELAND SECURITY: FIGHTING TERRORISM SINCE 1492, and I'D RATHER BE SMASHING IMPERIALISM. He popped off the top. It was filled with clones: marijuana-speak for cuttings. He said, "Uncle Timmy to the rescue."

The strains he brought were all developed in the cannabis culture of northern California.

There was Trainwreck. As a stoner review put it: "A Humboldt classic that takes off like a rocket, and powers you into an outer orbit. Look for body sensations. This pot is known among the club scene as one that will definitely not couch-lock you, but leave you energetic enough to go all night. Definitely not for insomnia, but works great for PTSD and chronic pain. Very good for depression. Too energetic for some, but thrill seekers will be satisfied."

And there was Granddaddy Purple, which, since the plants are female, should really be called Grandmother Purple. "My word for this stoner weed is clarity. Expect a clear high with lots of clarity and easy introspection. And then expect to fall asleep."

And Afwreck. "A cross of Afghani and Trainwreck. The high is more of a creeper, and on the mellow end. It's a daily driver, if peace and joy are your thing. This strain reliably reminds me why I started smoking pot. I haven't enjoyed smoking this much since the bags of gold Colombian I used to get from a guy named Dharma. Fun, fun, fun."

*

He was right. Better strains made a big difference. There's a cliché hiding in there somewhere, perhaps about silk purses and sow's ears, but despite my recent ingestion of some Grandmother Purple I can't seem to find the clarity to put it together. Besides, I'm getting pretty sleepy.

Better strains don't cure stupidity.

My first grow was outside. That in itself is not stupid. Nor is it stupid to live near the ocean in a temperate redwood rainforest. What is stupid is to plant sun-loving plants under a thick canopy of rain- and fog-loving redwoods, for fear that if I planted them in a meadow, Feds in helicopters would spot my measly half-dozen plants and mount a major SWAT operation to "take me down."

The mold *Botrytis* loves damp conditions, and it loves cannabis. Consequently, my first grow led to medium-sized marijuana plants that were no longer green but covered crown to soil with fuzzy brown-gray mold. My first solution? To run an extension cord from my house to the plants and hook up a fan to, I don't know, dry off the plants, blow off the *Botrytis*? It didn't work. My next solution was to try the exact same thing again the next year. Surprisingly, that didn't work either.

If I were a normal pot grower, I would now tell you stories about the fifteen pounds of *Botrytis* I harvested . . .

This was when Tim and Mario intervened. Mario built me a grow room. When the electrician he brought with him—a four hour drive each way, since you can't trust just any ol' electrician—was done, he told me the room was rated for 7000 watts. I bought myself twelve 600-watt lights, and was surprised when the circuit breakers flipped. The stupidity is not that despite my degree in physics, I evidently couldn't figure out that 600 X 12 > 7000. The stupidity also isn't that after the breakers repeatedly flipped, I still didn't do the math. The stupidity is that I called the electrician, who drove all the way down, walked into the grow room, counted the lights, looked at me a long moment, then did the math out loud.

Then came the fertilizer fiasco. Because the soil I bought consisted of "composted forest humus, sphagnum peat moss, perlite, earthworm castings, bat guano, humic acid, oyster shell, and dolomite lime," and because ad copy for the soil said it was "alive with beneficial microbes and fungi that help break down organic matter and feed the plant roots," I somehow concluded this meant I didn't have to feed the plants anything else.[1]

And then I was surprised when the buds were small.

At least I didn't water them four times a day.

Idiocy loves company, so I asked a friend what was the stupidest thing he did when he was first growing. He responded, "You mean besides almost burning down my house? I converted a spare bedroom to a grow scene, and evidently my circuit breakers weren't doing their job, because I soon noticed a terrible smell. I turned off the electricity, put on a headlamp, got a screwdriver, unscrewed the wall plates, and took out the junction boxes. Behind most of them the wire insulation had melted. The interiors of the walls were scorched and smoking."

I asked another friend— someone who has been growing since the early nineties—who said, "Oh, the stories I could tell you. During the early days of cannabis liberalization, after Prop 215 passed, those who hustled weed as a side gig to make a little money and subsidize their smoking habit realized they could make a lot more money if they grew the weed. Prop 215 created a legal grey area that provided growers with a sense of security from the state—and with indoor pot fetching upwards of $4,000 a pound, indoor operations exploded. Just about anyone with access to a spare room or garage set up a room. And hundreds of people moved to the Emerald Triangle to grow. Some loved the plants, some saw liberation from wage labor through cannabis cultivation. Some succeeded. Many failed. Some were too busy or too inexperienced to do it right, and others were too stupid and lazy.

---

[1] Just yesterday I went to a marijuana forum and saw a post by a new grower who thought the same thing I used to, and was using the same soil! Ah, sweet summer child.

Some basically wanted to find a way to smoke weed and play computer games all day.

"We always joked that you could identify a shitty grower by looking at the condition of the house plants. Most shitty growers couldn't grow a house plant, nor could they tell the difference between a tomato and a poison ivy.

"There was this one East Coaster I knew who set up a scene. He was a good guy, working class, a cook who moved to Humboldt chasing a lady. He rented a room in a house from an older guy who had a medical card. So they got to thinking they could make some money setting up a scene. But other than the mold in the fridge, they couldn't keep shit alive. The first few rounds they struggled with mites, over-fertilizing, underwatering—you name it. Then about six weeks into their next round the plants got powdery mildew. They'd read in some cannabis book that burning sulfur for an hour keeps powdery mildew at bay. So he went to the grow store, bought the sulfur and the burners, then hung them in the room. He covered all the lights with cardboard to protect them from the sulfur dust, lit the burners, and went into the living room. He started to smoke a joint, and halfway through he got a call from work. A waiter had called in sick and they needed him to get into the restaurant ASAP to cover the waiter's four-to-nine shift. Half-baked, the guy said okay, grabbed his shit, and split to work. At seven, he got a call from his housemate. The grow room was on fire and the fire department was on its way. Before he'd left the house, he'd forgotten to tell his housemate to take off the cardboard. Luckily, he got no jail time—the Prop 215 license became a literal get-out-of-jail-free card—but half the house was destroyed. He and his crew rebuilt and tried for the next two years to turn a profit.

"And one more story. A professional couple in their fifties owned some land and outbuildings in the hills. They asked an experienced grower to build and run a ten-light scene for them. They worked out the financials, and he set it up in an outbuilding next to the main house. Then in mid-July, about four weeks from completing the first run, the couple's out-of-town retired parents made an unexpected visit. Fearing the parents would hear the loud humming of the ventilation system, one of them rushed to the grow room and shut off the fans. The parents and the couple had a wonderful rest of the day, wandering around their property. The temperature was in the nineties, and you know how hot lights are. The grower showed up that night to water, and of course found that all the plants had baked to death."

You start with seeds that came hidden in a box of sweets or that you got from some guy, or you start with clones given you by a friend. You plant them in your favorite soil, whether you purchased that soil or it's a special blend you mix yourself in a small pot; small so, as your mother tells you, the tiny plants don't get discouraged by too much root space. As the plants grow, you transplant them into larger pots, then larger pots again. You tell them how beautiful they are and you thank them.

Cannabis is a "short-day obligate photoperiodic" species: a fancy way of saying it blooms when days shorten below a certain length. Lots of plants bloom based on the number of hours of light (or dark) they receive. Long-day obligate plants—normally early-season plants—bloom when daylight hours pass a certain length. Short-day obligate plants bloom when the hours of light fall below a certain threshold.

What this means is that when you grow marijuana indoors, you run your lights around eighteen hours per day to "veg," that is, grow the plants in a pre-bloom stage; and then when you want them to bloom, you reduce that time to about twelve hours per day. It makes sense, then, to have at least two rooms, so you can always have one room vegging while the other blooms.

If you hold plants back in the veg room, you can keep them alive more or less forever. Some people do this to keep "mothers," and from these mothers continually make new plants by cloning. But since mothers take up space, some growers don't bother with them, instead making a few clones off the plants they want to keep before they put the plants into the bloom room.

Just like humans aren't capable of reproducing until they reach puberty, a short photoperiod won't cause seedlings to bloom. This makes sense, because in nature, baby short-day obligate plants need time to germinate in the long nights of early spring prior to blooming. Only when the plants reach a certain age do they, too, become capable of reproduction, which is, after all, a primary point of flowers.

Clones, however, are the same age as the mother (or, if for some reason you want to clone a male, the father). This means you could, if you wanted to, bloom them immediately. This also means that some lines of plants run back decades. Some of mine run back almost two decades that I know of, and who knows how long before then.

So you grow the plants to the size you want them (mine are usually about six feet tall when I flip them, although most people flip them much sooner) and then move the plants to the bloom room—again telling them how beautiful they are and thanking them for gracing you with their presence—where you can witness the miracle of sexual maturity. In the first week, the plants stretch, some strains by up to 30 percent. Between the first and second week you can see tiny white stigmata—hairlike strands—start to grow where soon there will be flowers. From the second to third week, the flowers develop into small buds covered with these stigmata. Each week, the buds get larger, with some buds growing together into larger and larger colas (some people's—not mine—as big as baseball bats!). Weeks five through seven show explosive bud growth. Toward the end, the stigmata turn red or brown, one indicator of full maturity.

Another (the primary) indicator is visible through a magnifier. The buds are covered with "trichomes." Trichomes—and this may be a surprise to many in marijuana-world—are not unique to marijuana. They're simply small, often hair-like structures. The word *trichome* comes from a root meaning "hair"—on plants, algae, lichen, and protists. They have all sorts of shapes and purposes on different species. The trichomes on bean leaves, for example, can impale the "feet"—tarsi to entomologists and pedants—of insects. Trichomes on other plants can prevent herbivores from feeding, either by harming or physically preventing small creatures from getting to the plant itself, or by making the leaves irritable to larger herbivore's palates. (Think stinging nettles:

the sting comes from chemicals on the tips of trichomes). Trichomes can also keep frost away from the surface cells of plants. They can act like tiny forests and reduce wind speed at the plant, reducing water loss. They can catch droplets of water from fog for the plant to drink. Venus flytraps have three types of trichomes on their traps: one secretes a substance that attracts insects; another, when disturbed by an insect, triggers the trap to close; and the third secretes enzymes to digest the insect and then absorb the digested materials. Likewise, sundews are known for their large trichomes that attract, trap, and digest insects.

And then there's marijuana trichomes. They're small resin glands on buds and some leaves that look like frosting. Magnified they look like cylinders with a sphere atop each one, like so many tiny mushrooms. These trichomes—the major sources of the cannabinoids for which marijuana is famous—are clear until soon before harvest. As the plant matures the trichomes cloud. If you want to wait longer to harvest, the cloudiness will change from white to yellow to reddish. The different colors provide different effects when ingested.

Most plants take seven to ten weeks of blooming to mature. I've got a couple of strains that go as short as six-and-a-half weeks, and one that goes as long as fifteen.

When it's time to harvest, you again tell them they're beautiful, and again you thank them, and this time you wish them Godspeed on the next part of their story.

How different the world must seem to those whose sense of smell is more acute than ours, which means to almost everyone: dogs, bears, elephants, sharks, salmon, snakes, tortoises, vultures, moths, wasps, ants, and—if by "sense of smell" we mean ability to perceive and differentiate between chemicals in air or water, and not more narrowly the binding of molecules to olfactory receptors—many plants.

I'm standing at the edge of a redwood forest. I see scores of shades of green, from the light green of new shoots of grass to the purpled green of more mature blades; from the varied greens of redwood needles to the just as varied greens of alder or cascara leaves. And it's not just green. It's the dark rust-ish color of the duff, the yellow and black of fallen leaves and of the camouflaged banana slugs who hide among and eat them. It's the myriad browns of soil, of barks.

The world is just as rich, complex, and exquisitely layered for those with strong senses of smell as it is for those of us who are more visually-oriented. Just as you or I might be drawn to movement or bright colors, scents can draw those who rely on smell. Salmon in the middle of the ocean smell the stream where they began and find their way home. Insects eat plants, who release scents detected by predator insects who come to feed. Elephants smell water a dozen miles away.

Someone once dumped a freezer at a friend's house, and another friend and I were going to use my pickup to haul it to the waste transfer station. Inside the unplugged yet sealed freezer was some very old meat. We popped the top and staggered backwards from the smell. But there were two cool things: 1) within a couple of minutes, scores of flies arrived, when we'd seen none before; and 2) within ten minutes, a vulture arrived to circle overhead, when once again we'd seen none before.

Within six hundred seconds, molecules of rotting meat had floated hundreds of feet into the sky and had been carried beyond the tree-shortened horizon to this vulture, who smelled the meat—although the scent was diluted into billions of cubic feet of air—then quickly determined the location of the food and flew the distance to claim it.

Which brings us to pot. Often, the first thing that comes to mind when people think of marijuana is the smell. Sweet, skunky, piney funk. Just those four words will give most stoners a goofy smile. The smells are our noses responding to chemicals, called terpenes, emitted by the plants. Terpenes are what make lemon, pine, lavender, mint, hops, pot, and others smell like they do. And pot shares many of these terpenes. Limonene is also found in lemons, alpha-pinene is also found in pine needles, linalool is also made by lavender, and the skunk smell probably comes from myrcene, also made by hops (and wild thyme) but, interestingly enough, not by skunks.

CHAPTER 3

Beginnings

I asked Tim about his first experience with marijuana culture.

He thought a moment, then said, "Back in the eighties college was still reasonably-priced, so by working part time during the school year and two jobs in the summer, I finished college with more money than when I started. Point being I wasn't, like so many kids these days, indentured on graduation. So after college I kicked around the country while I figured out what I wanted to do. I ended up in a hostel in San Francisco, where I got to know this guy who was hustling pot. One time he said he was going to make a run to southern Humboldt to pick up some weed and asked if I wanted to go along. I said sure.

"We headed up in his beater. I didn't find out till we were on the way that the car had no license plate, that he had a shotgun under a blanket in the back seat, and that he was a convicted felon. But by then it was too late for me to bail.

"We went up 101 to Humboldt, turned off on a paved road, turned off on a dirt road, and kept driving on this winding road till we came to a big open field where I saw four hippies sitting on chairs in the backs of a couple of pickups, smoking joints, taking hits from four-foot canisters of what I later learned was nitrous oxide, and shooting at abandoned cars."

I stared at him.

"They had big garbage bags full of marijuana. It was like a small farmer's market, only here the sellers were shooting guns while stoned off their asses on weed and nitrous oxide."

I started to ask, "If that was your first experience with marijuana culture, why—"

"My second was even worse. The next spring this same guy asked me to help him start his garden. I've always loved plants, so, despite that first trip, I said yes. We drove up. This time in a pickup. But same lack of a license plate. Same felon in possession of a firearm. Only this time the back was filled with bags of potting soil, along with his motocross motorcycle. And in the cab he had this weird paper that looked like a page of postage stamps, with all sorts of funky pictures of Disney characters on it. I'd never seen anything like it. I looked at it pretty closely and put it down. It ends up it was LSD, which I'd never even seen, much less used. I later learned you can't get high from just touching blotter LSD, but it was 90 degrees in the pickup—with of course no air conditioning—and I was sweaty. I must have touched the paper, got it wet, touched my lips . . . ." He shook his head, blew out a breath through pursed lips, and continued, "So he drove way back in the forest somewhere and stopped at a trailhead. We got out. He pulled out the motorcycle, and we put bags of soil between us and in front of him. He drove a deer trail till the undergrowth got so thick the motorcycle got stuck. Then we had to carry the bags one by one about a mile up the trail to the site of his guerrilla grow. He walked faster than I did, so we got separated. I was walking back from dropping off the first bag when the LSD kicked in, and I started hearing airplane spotters flying low overhead, and after that, helicopters. I even saw a cop riding a horse. I was sure the feds had sussed us. Of course, later I learned there were no planes and no helicopters. Why would the feds do overflights that early in the season? It's nuts. The only thing that was flying was me. Anyway, I dove into the undergrowth and crawled away. I was seeing cops everywhere, on horses, on foot, rappelling out of trees. I hid under the bushes so long that mice started crawling over my hands—at least I thought mice started crawling over my hands, but I'm no longer sure the mice were any more real than the cops. It started getting late, and I started to get scared not only of these phantom police but also of a non-phantom, cold, spring night. I needed to make it back to the truck, but I couldn't take the trail because of my paranoia. So I headed cross-country and soon became lost. I couldn't make any noise because

I was scared of the police I was still convinced were there. I came across a house, but I couldn't go up and talk to them because I was sure they were in on the massive fed raid. Finally, I somehow came across the road we drove up on, right when my acquaintance was driving by on his motorcycle. He was really pissed: 'You were going to help me carry soil! I spent the whole afternoon looking for you.' It ends up that the house belonged to friends of his, and they'd all considered calling search and rescue to find me but didn't because then search and rescue—and more broadly, cops—might have found their grows. 'We didn't know what to do,' he said, 'so we didn't do anything. We figured you were toast, man.'"

I gave my head a quick shake, and finally finished my question: "Given those introductions, why did you want anything to do with marijuana culture?"

"Because not all of it is that bad. Some of it is great. It's this really odd mix. And in some ways, it's not really accurate to talk about cannabis culture at all. It's more accurate to talk about cultures, plural. The illegality made mass culture and mass communication much more difficult, with communication taking place mainly in person and silly codes over the telephone."

I could imagine some of these coded conversations: "How are your tomatoes doing?" "Great! My tomato blossoms are the size of coke bottles. And yours?" "Baseball bats." "Oh, did I say coke bottles? I meant fire hydrants."

He continued, "So various cultures sprang up throughout the region. Marijuana culture might be different in Whitethorn than Petrolia, Petrolia than Honeydew, Southern Humboldt than Mendocino or Trinity counties. But even those differences aren't as great as the differences over time."

I knew that the person to talk to about the history of cannabis culture was my friend Tony, the coauthor of this book. We spoke on the back porch of his home in McKinleyville, just north of Arcata. As well as being a professor of sociology at Humboldt State University and a long-time grassroots environmentalist, he's a founding faculty member of the Humboldt Institute for Interdisciplinary Marijuana Research. He also coaches and plays lacrosse. As we talked, he taught me how to use a lacrosse stick to throw a ball for his dog. My back got tired of this long before his dog did.

He said, between throws, "Cannabis culture in northern California emerged in the late 1960s, during the countercultural revolution, when there was a mass movement of mainly educated, young, white urbanites leaving mainstream society in pursuit of an alternative lifestyle and coming to the Pacific Northwest, specifically the Emerald Triangle. It was here that they formed communes and homesteads on these landscapes in Northern California."

He tossed the ball. His dog retrieved it, dropped it at his feet. He scooped it, twirled the stick, tossed it again.

"You have to remember," he said, "that these landscapes had been devastated by almost a century of industrial logging, mining, and agriculture, so land was abundant and cheap. These new settlers didn't come here to grow weed. They came here to attempt to live a different lifestyle. And with them, they brought different cultural values, values that were countermaterialist—or nonmaterialist, if you will. They valued things like simplicity, freedom, closeness to nature. This was all based in an explicit rejection of the values of the mainstream culture, which many found morally bankrupt, and in response to the anti-ecological practices of industrial society."

I asked how this specifically affected their relationship to cannabis.

He said, "The back-to-the-landers brought cannabis with them as part of their lifestyle. And the important thing to keep in mind is that they were already disillusioned with traditional concepts of authority and legality. They didn't find meaning in obeying laws they didn't believe in. In other words, they had no problem with illegal activities, so in this worldview growing cannabis wasn't a big deal."

The dog brought back the ball. Tony scooped it, tossed it to me. I didn't catch it, but at least I knocked it down. I tried scooping, eventually had to put my foot in front of the ball to keep it from rolling away. The dog panted, ran back and forth between me and Tony. I tossed the ball. Or tried to. I spiked it. The dog grabbed it anyway, on its first high bounce.

Tony said, "The historian Ray Raphael writes about early marijuana culture in his book *Cash Crop*, where he talks about a 'traditional rural anarchy'[1] that already pervaded this sparsely populated region in which these new settlers arrived. This was a culture that distrusted authority and the mainstream notion of 'the rule of law.' And the new settlers especially loved cannabis. They cultivated it in their gardens, primarily for personal consumption. They didn't grow it to make money. They viewed it in a way as a form of political protest, as people of that generation talk about. All of this was facilitated by their remote, rural geography where there was little, if any, law enforcement."

I asked, "What year are we up to by now?"

"The seventies. Which means we have to talk about the War on Drugs. At that point a lot of marijuana was coming into the United States through its southern border. So the United States increased enforcement against smuggling at the border[2] and pressured Mexico to increase efforts to eradicate the growing of both opium poppies and marijuana. In 1975 the United States started assisting these efforts through supplying helicopters and lots of herbicides, primarily paraquat and 2,4-D. American scientists started finding these chemicals in pot here in the US.

"The US government was forced to put together a public health campaign to let people know they shouldn't smoke cannabis from Mexico because it had paraquat in it. Of course, this had the desired effect of people not wanting to smoke Mexican weed, but the demand for weed didn't change. The sourcing just shifted from Mexico to Jamaica and Colombia. So it didn't stop people from consuming cannabis at all; it just shifted the country of origin."

He tossed me the ball again. This time I almost caught it, and this time I was able to at least get the ball off the porch.

---

[1] Ray Raphael, *Cash Crop: An American Dream* (Casper, CA: Ridge Times Press, 1985), 36.

[2] You might think the phrase "smuggling at the border" is redundant, but planes, boats, and even submarines as well as parcel delivery services are used to smuggle.

He continued, "Cannabis studies geographer Dominic Corva calls this the balloon effect: when you squeeze a balloon, the air has to go somewhere, and that's the effect of supply-side interdictions on the southern border. The supply chain shifted to where there was no pressure."

"How," I asked, "does this relate to California cannabis culture?"

"The back-to-the-landers were already growing and smoking cannabis but not really selling it to make a living. They had this spiritual connection to the plant; for many, it was sacred medicine, not a market commodity. But federal government interdiction efforts and the paraquat scare artificially inflated the price, from maybe $200/lb. in the early seventies to over $2,000/lb. Suddenly, weed was worth selling. These prohibitionist efforts essentially acted like a farm aid program for northern California growers, leading to the emergence of a cottage industry where it became rational to not just grow your own 'headstash' but to grow a bit more to pay your bills. And some of these growers traveled to Thailand, India, Pakistan, Afghanistan, and elsewhere to get seeds—the very best genetics they could find—to grow here.

"Now we need to bring in another set of actors. Remember that the economy of northern California was primarily extractive—mainly timber—which means it experienced boom-and-bust cycles. As we head into the eighties, we had locals who were hit hard by the decline of the timber industry: timberland owners, loggers, mill workers, ranchers, and rural laborers. They also started turning to cannabis. Ray Raphael calls them 'the pragmatists': When the economy is in the shitter, and you don't have a way to feed your family, what do you do? Well, if you live in rural northern California, you might grow some weed.

"At this point you basically had two different marijuana cultures in the same place, with two very different relationships to the plant. You had the eco-groovy 'we're not in it for materialist values—we're in it for lifestyle or spiritual reasons' back-to-the-landers, and you had the pragmatists with attitudes and practices reminiscent of industrial agricultural communities.

"Then to make it even more complicated, you had a third category coming into the mix: the 'green-rushers'—opportunists who moved in because they saw there was a lot of money to be made. I don't like to use the terms 'organized crime' or 'cartels,' but I'm comfortable saying that the back-to-the-landers and to a certain extent the locals pumped money back into communities, using proceeds from the sale of cannabis to put together community centers, health centers, radio stations. They addressed the needs of rural communities that the state failed to address. They helped build infrastructures in rural communities that might not have had them in the past. The new green-rushers didn't have these ties to communities and in many cases had no interest in developing these ties. And, of course, since they came here specifically to make money, their land practices mirrored the model of industrial agriculture. Many of these green-rushers not only had no ties to the community, they didn't even live here. They just bought land and, like feudal lords, farmed everything out, raking in the money.

"By now we're into the eighties, which also means we're well-past the half-assed War on Drugs of the seventies. Reagan really took off the gloves by increasing fines and penalties for those caught growing cannabis and by putting into place laws like the Comprehensive Crime and Control Act of 1984. He introduced mandatory minimum sentences for marijuana as well as asset forfeiture, whereby law enforcement could seize property—land, vehicles, whatever—they deemed to have been associated with the growth or distribution of marijuana and, of course, other drugs. At the same time, the antidrug California attorney general was putting together a program called CAMP—Campaign Against Marijuana Planting—that was a joint effort between federal, state, county, and municipal governments aimed at eradicating cultivation and trafficking in cannabis. So you have armed paramilitary units converging on rural communities from the air and land. Think for a second about sitting on your back porch, enjoying your late summer afternoon with your children, when all of a sudden a military helicopter is hovering above you, then a bunch of heavily armed men converge on you and your family. This was CAMP, and it terrorized rural cannabis communities for almost two decades."

I said, not entirely seriously, "I always thought their money would have been more effectively spent flying helicopters over grows and scattering pollen from male marijuana plants all over the region. It would have effectively ruined a lot of crops at no cost to the environment."

He laughed half-heartedly, which is probably what the joke was worth, then continued, "Prior to CAMP, police intervention had been, even under Reagan, a bit of a slow trickle. There was no concerted effort by local law enforcement to eradicate weed. But then in came CAMP, and all hell broke loose.

"Everybody in the weed game recognized they had to do things differently. No longer could they plant in the full sun in open gardens. So they started planting where spotters in helicopters couldn't see, in the shade in forests.

"Another side effect from all of these laws is that a lot of these grows started moving onto public lands. If forfeiture laws make it so the feds can seize your land if you're growing some weed—even if you owned the land outright long before you grew any marijuana for sale—then it becomes a rational decision to grow on someone else's land, in this case on public lands. People would go cut trees on National Forest land, use herbicides and pesticides, pump water from salmon-bearing streams for irrigation. It turned into a fucking mess. At first those public land growers were twenty plants here, thirty plants there, but in the eighties there were thousands of plant grows doing real damage to ecosystems. Putting out rodenticides to kill mice, and then as a result killing all the predators who ate those mice. These for the most part weren't the back-to-the-landers—who were as appalled by this as you or I—but were the pragmatists, the green-rushers, and the children of the back-to-the-landers."

"Their kids?"

"In many ways, the second generation of back-to-the-landers didn't make the same choices as their parents. They were born here, didn't flee the city, didn't flee the Vietnam War. And though they shared their parents' distrust of authority—after all, they saw their families being terrorized by these paramilitary groups—the rest of their values—ecological, social, and communal—didn't necessarily coincide with their parents'. It's no secret they often lacked the same land ethic and morality as their parents. They were often much more money-oriented as well in their relationship to growing marijuana.

"What really changed things was that when the kids started to get into their teens, the parents recognized that if the kids got busted growing weed at fourteen, they'd just get slapped on the wrist. They wouldn't be sent to prison, because they're kids. This meant that a lot of these kids got involved in the industry in their early teens. The hope of the parents was that the kids would save and go to college. But this ended up being naïve."

"How so?"

"A lot of these kids thought, 'Who needs college if we're making all this money?' So the much higher price for pot ended up giving these kids an economic incentive that changed their cultural and ecological practices. They weren't light on the land. They grew too much. They used pesticides and fertilizers.

"I can't overemphasize how harmful the War on Drugs and CAMP have been to cannabis culture. That shift away from the more ecological and communal perspective to a more industrial model didn't happen in isolation. It never does. As a result of these CAMP helicopters flying overhead, growers were pushed inside, giving us diesel dope."

"Diesel dope?"

"Weed grown indoors with lights and fans powered by large industrial generators run on diesel. And, of course, that's a result of the price cannabis was fetching in the market because of prohibition, upwards of $2,000 a pound in the eighties. You have that fear of jail and forfeiture and the economic engine of prohibition incentivizing people to grow indoors, which is ecologically far worse than growing in the sun outside."

By then I could throw the ball at least well enough to make the dog work. I couldn't aim at all, though, and not infrequently the ball ended up in a huge bunch of tall grass. The dog didn't seem to mind and would dive in till we had disappearing dog, only to pop out several seconds later, ball in mouth and tail wagging.

Tony said, "There's another group I need to mention: the trimmigrants."

"Trimmigrants?"

"Yeah, they've always been here, since the beginnings of the commercial cannabis culture. They are people who come from around the world and work on people's farms to harvest and trim weed."

"I've heard about that," I say. "People from Ireland or Germany or Australia or Japan who say it's always been on their bucket list to come to northern California to trim, which—given what hard work harvesting and trimming are—seems kind of strange."

"That might be because you live here, and if you want to hang out with marijuana plants you just have to walk out to your or someone else's grow space. That's not an option for people in a lot of places around the world. It's more than that, though. Coming to northern California to experience the cannabis scene is like going to the south of France for wine or, for some people, like going to see the Sistine Chapel or Yankee Stadium. Or maybe it's like it was for those back-to-the-landers to go to Central Asia back in the day. This is the Holy Land for cannabis connoisseurs.

"In any case, the trimmigrants are an interesting group. At first most of the trimmers were friends and families of growers, a close-knit group of people who came back every year. And then in the 1990s the market expanded and there was a need for more labor than just your friends and family. Not to mention that your friends and family were also growing weed and making enough money that they didn't need to sit at a table for ten hours a day trimming cannabis. So these folks came to the area filling a need for labor. And they have some of the cultural values of the back-to-the-landers. A lot of them are travelers. They certainly aren't materialist. They could live out of a backpack and be relatively happy."

"What year are we up to now?" I asked.

Tony responded, "Let's move to the 1990s, and to Proposition 215 in 1996, which legalized growing in California for medical purposes. Of course, marijuana is helpful for quite a few medical conditions, but nobody can deny that a lot of people used this legal cover to grow for sale."

"I have a long-time stoner friend," I said, "who thinks the whole medical marijuana movement was a trojan horse for recreational legalization."

"Marijuana has helped a lot of people with their pain and other symptoms of their diseases, and indeed the diseases themselves," he responded, "which doesn't alter the fact that Prop 215 brought a whole new crowd of people into the cannabis culture mix. You had, for example, Humboldt State graduates who'd done a bit of trimming as students and who enjoyed spending their summers doing things like attending the music festival *Reggae on the River*. A lot of them saw the money they could make and the lifestyle weed could support, so they started growing. And it wasn't just kids from Humboldt. They came from all over. I'd say most weren't really environmentally conscious and didn't have any connection to the back-to-the-land movement or any background in agriculture. They also didn't have a connection to the green-rushers. They just liked getting high and listening to reggae and bluegrass. Think of it like frat-boy culture but centered around cannabis instead of beer. Replace keg stands with huge glass bongs and you've about got it. A lot of their lives revolved around smoking high-octane cannabis, getting as high as possible, and spending money like you can't believe. Throwing it all over the place. Which was pretty easy to do when in 1996 you were getting $4,000 a pound. Anyone with half a brain can make a lot of money on that.

"And they didn't just sell cannabis. They were selling coke, heroin, ecstasy, LSD. Nothing was off-limits. They weren't into cannabis to help their community but rather for individualistic, selfish reasons. Many were just hedonists who wanted to make a boatload of money and get really fucked up. Unfortunately, many of these types of growers became big players in the push for complete legalization, which is one reason it has been such a disaster for traditional cannabis communities. They're basically just regular capitalists."

"On drugs."

"Yeah, on drugs, like a lot of the other capitalists."

I threw the ball. The dog retrieved it. I was getting better, but I was also starting to notice muscles in my back I didn't know existed. Tomorrow I was going to pay for this conversation.

Tony asked me what else I wanted to know about cannabis culture.

I said, "I hear what you're saying about the degradation of traditional marijuana culture over the last few decades. But despite these changes I still know some people who are using this as a cottage industry. I know some artists who grow to support their art. I knew some tree sitters who said they routinely received anonymous envelopes full of cash clearly from growers who wanted to support them in the frontline work. I did a benefit one time for a couple of eco-activists down in Garberville. This was in fact my introduction to marijuana culture. I knew nothing about it before then. I just knew that the activists had asked me to do a benefit, and so I did it for free. I drove down, went to the venue, and saw all these people in dirty coveralls walking in and putting five or six hundred-dollar bills in the donation basket. Because I'm not very bright sometimes, it took me about ten minutes to twig to what was going on."

"That's an important piece. We tend to think of cannabis culture in isolation, but you have to remember that from the 1980s through the 1990s northern California was in the midst of these intense timber wars, where MAXXAM/Pacific Lumber was clearcutting ancient redwoods, and a huge resistance movement rose up against it. Grassroots environmentalism emerged during the 1980s on the West Coast and the Pacific Northwest. It also happened to be in the heart of the pre-existing cannabis culture. So it really is true that at least some of the cannabis growers funded a lot of the resistance to MAXXAM/Pacific Lumber and, indeed, a lot of environmentalism in the region. I don't know if this is the right way to frame it, but the environmental movement funded by cannabis really flourished in the nineties. Cannabis also helped fund and spark a lot of the resistance around the WTO during that decade as well.

"So you're right. The influence of cannabis culture on the environmental and social justice movements cannot be overstated, especially given the prices cannabis was fetching throughout that time. Some growers used the money to buy expensive cars, coke, and guns; some used it to support themselves so they could engage in environmental activism; and some used it to fund movements and lawsuits, and to buy land to protect it.

"I really need to emphasize that at the time the state was absent from these rural communities. During the timber boom it was absent in terms of regulating the timber industry; they let the timber industry do what it wanted. When the back-to-the-landers moved in there, they had to not only repair prior ecological damage but to create their own social service institutions as well. And they funded it with cannabis. You have community centers that provided free lunches to children and the homeless, health centers, radio stations, schools, and environmental organizations that never could have been created without money from cannabis. I've talked to numerous folks who would dedicate portions of their farms to different causes, a kind of cannabis tithing: 'This plant is dedicated to the school, while the proceeds from this plant are dedicated to the radio station.' This was a common practice in traditional cannabis communities in the eighties and nineties."

"Can you bring us up-to-date?"

"Yes, Clinton was pretty hands-off, wasn't as obsessed with cannabis as were previous administrations. And I think, post Prop 215, the writing was really on the wall for eventual legalization."

"Which was my stoner friend's point."

"When legalization became a real possibility, there was a huge uptick in interest by those with shedloads of money. As we've seen, cannabis culture has been from the beginning molded by governmental policies, whether these policies are prohibitionist or regular old capitalist. How people grow is influenced by how the state works. And the state has really focused on megagrowers. So in 2012 Oregon legalized it. Washington legalized it. California began anticipating it. There was—and continues to be—another green rush, this one not primarily individuals but capitalists. Entrepreneurs and speculators. People in the finance and tech industries looking for places to invest."

"Huge alcohol companies. Agribusiness."

"You name it. And in response to this we have small farm trade associations developing, trying their best to keep the cottage industries alive (of course some of these trade associations have themselves been co-opted by Big Canna and no longer serve the interests of small growers). Which is pretty much where we are today. Things look bad for small farms in the face of what the state and capitalism does, but there are those who are still hanging on."

CHAPTER 4

A Growing Relationship

For me, the hardest part of growing is harvesting. That would be equally true if I farmed rabbits. And while cell death in both plants and animals occurs when cells don't receive energy and materials necessary to survive, in plants this generally happens more slowly. In other words, it generally takes longer for doomed plants to die.

I think about this each time I harvest a plant. Honestly, I think about this each time I eat.

After you choose plants to harvest—thanking them, as I mentioned before—you remove all of the big leaves, normally called "fan leaves." Some people remove them when the plants are still growing, but I generally presume plants know better than I what they need, so I don't remove them till it's time to harvest. Often, people put these leaves in compost piles or worm bins (worms love them), and people with stealth grows in cities may put them in garbage bags and toss them in public dumpsters. I spoke with one grower who said, "I give them to my chickens. They *love* them. And have you ever seen a pig eat fan leaves? It's the cutest thing. I worked at a farm where we fed the leaves to the pigs, and those were the happiest pigs I've ever seen, rolling around, snorting happily together, so precious."

I juice them, and drink the juice for my Crohn's disease. It's the primary way I consume cannabis.

My Prop 215 doctor told me she wanted me to drink a full glass of this per day. As much as this juice helps my Crohn's, there are at least three reasons I can't do that much.

The first is that the taste is vile. Given a choice between dying an agonizing death and having to drink a glass of this stuff every day, I'd have to think long and hard. Or maybe flip a coin. It's like the joke where one old man asks the other how his cold bath cure for rheumatism is going, and the other responds, "I got rid of my rheumatism, but now I've got cold baths."

My niece is a practitioner of Chinese Traditional Medicine, trained in China. Once I complained to her about the taste. She smelled it, had a sip, and started laughing.

I asked what was so funny.

"Yeah, this is bad," she responded, "but you haven't tasted vile till you've had some of the traditional Chinese prescriptions. One of the worst is Sheng Hua Teng, or Birth Cleaning Soup. After childbirth it helps your uterus contract back to size and helps you stop bleeding sooner."

"How bad is it?"

She laughed again. "I don't remember. That's the wonderful thing about childbirth. Directly after labor and delivery your brain washes itself in all these chemicals, so you forget the pain. (You also spend the next six months to a year in a brain fog.) This benefits humankind because if you remembered what it felt like, you'd never do it again. So, in the middle of the next labor your brain kicks in and says, 'Oh yeah, I remember this. This is horrible. I can't believe I have to do this again.' Because the Sheng Hua Tang is taken directly after giving birth, I always forget how nasty it is until I have to drink it again, and then I remember, oh my goodness, this stuff is awful. It's retch-inducing and I have to drink it every day for a week."

I said, "You convinced me."

"That marijuana juice isn't vile?" she responded.

"No," I said, "Never to give birth."

The second is that it takes a lot of leaves to produce not much juice. In order to get that much juice, I'd have to harvest ten or so plants a day. For a solo grower, that's a lot of plants.

And gosh, what would I do with all of those buds?

The third is that if I drank that much juice I'd be more or less constantly stoned. I guess on the good side, if I drank that much I probably wouldn't care—and might not even notice—that I was dying an agonizing death.

I know we've all been told that THC—tetrahydrocannabinol, the primary psychoactive chemical in marijuana—has to be heated to work, but I can tell you from experience that either a) it doesn't have to be heated, or b) the juice contains so much THC that heating isn't necessary.

I didn't know that the first time I drank juice.

I'd bought a fancy juicer—it has to be a wheatgrass juicer, not a cheap one—and processed enough leaves to fill half a glass. It was seven in the evening. I was at my mom's house. She complained about the awful smell in her kitchen. This was a complaint she was to repeat every Saturday for the final thirteen years of her life, as I did my weekly juicing. Yes, it really does stink.

It tastes even worse.

Having been repeatedly reassured the juice wasn't psychoactive and having confirmed this on the internet—which meant it had to be true—I sipped it, almost retched, then seriously considered dumping the rest down the drain and throwing myself on the mercy of the gods and goddesses of Crohn's disease. But I gently reassured my gag reflex that after two big swallows this would all be over, and tossed it down the hatch.

For a while everything was fine. I started watching a baseball game with my mom.

After maybe an hour I got a dry mouth. A few minutes after that I thought for whatever reason I should mosey to the pantry. Potato chips seemed like a good idea. Half a bag later they still seemed like a good idea, in fact one of the best ideas I'd ever had. And somehow a funny idea too. My focus was by then very clear. I noticed—*was fixated on* works better—the texture of each chip as I watched someone's fingers—mine?—pulling them from the bag one by one, bringing them to my mouth. These hands seemed to be moving independently of me.

I wandered over to the peanut butter jar. Eating half the jar didn't seem like a good idea, but a half-dozen heaping spoonfuls sure did. And I'd never before noticed the perfect and delicate beauty left behind in the jar when you scoop out a spoonful of peanut butter: it's like eroded sandstone in the desert, only instant. And then I realized that never before in the history of humans eating peanut butter has there been precisely this set of large and small scallops. I had invented a form of sculpture, a form of performance art. I could take this show on the road, in museums and on street corners—each jar unique, each jar its own perfection.

This was followed by corn chips, then half of what remained of the potato chips, after which my hands decided to reach for a glass and the faucet and bring two big glasses of water up to my face. The water tasted better than anything I'd ever had, except for the potato chips, peanut butter, and corn chips. I ate a banana. It was just as good. I thought about having some ice cream, but decided not to, since I was on a diet.

But I did decide to write some poetry. It flowed like poop through a goose. I loved the poem even as I wrote it. Who knew poetry was so easy?

Here's the poem, to be read in poetry voice:

Standing in front of the open refrigerator

Still there two hours later

That's good bud.

I thought, in that moment (the next day I wasn't quite so sure), that this could easily net me that year's Frost Prize for best poem. I'd invented a poetry form, like Haiku, only without restrictions. Then it occurred to me that even better than a poem—no matter how wonderful that poem may be— would be an entire book of wonderful poems. And what would be a worthy topic for a serious book of wonderful poems? The insight came to me in a flash of marijuana-induced inspiration: classic rock songs with lyrics slightly altered to make the songs about cannabis. "Hotel California" would become a song about munchies. "More Than a Feeling" would be a song about your skeezy roommate stealing your pot ("It's more than just stealing, when I see Mary Jane walk away. I see my Mary Jane walking awaaaayyyyy."). Blue Öyster Cult would sing, "Don't Fear the Reefer." And the old coke ad would begin, "I'd like to build the world a home/and furnish it with buds/and cheesy fries and pizza pies/and chips made out of spuds.

. . ." Leaving aside the anachronism, I was amazed none of Whitman, Dickinson, or Plath ever thought of that. Their loss was my gain.

But I couldn't write those poems that night, because I couldn't remember which universe I was in. Was I in the universe where I was a writer, or did I dream that?

I wandered back to the sofa, watched some of the baseball game with my mom. This confused me even more. What mad universe was this, where the Seattle Mariners were winning?

It came time to go home. Still I sat, arms and legs weighing a hundred pounds each, and invisible plant fingers massaging the muscles of my back. The latter was nice, so I sat some more. Potato chips again seemed like a good idea. I got up. The bag was empty. I wasn't sure how that happened. The bag was full a while ago.

But, I thought, how long was a while ago? Ten minutes? An hour? A year? I stood, empty potato chip bag in one hand, spoon with mesmerizing smears of peanut butter in the other, thinking of mystery writer Ross MacDonald and his line about time passing slowly in "marijuana-fractured seconds."

I said good night to my mom and started home. The path from my mom's house to mine is three-eighths of a mile through a forest. In the previous six years I'd walked it more than 5,000 times. There are no side paths. Still, that night I got lost several times. I didn't panic, though. I was relaxed enough that I frequently considered lying down to take a nap, each time demurring only when I remembered the bears I'd seen in this forest. I kept walking.

The walk home took approximately 200 years.

After that, I learned to drink the juice only right before I go to bed. I drink maybe a fifth of a glass, the rest filled with orange juice.

It still tastes vile.

And I'm still never going to give birth.

Can you imagine how stoned a hot cup of marijuana would make someone? And can you imagine how bad that would taste?

*

I'm not sure why people pay money to get stoned. But a lot of people do.

Several years ago, I knew a woman who'd sold commercial quantities of hash in the early seventies. She said that, one time, she heard police sirens in the trailer park where she lived and became convinced the cops were coming for her, so to destroy evidence she ate her entire stash. Of course, the cops weren't coming for her. She told me she spent the weekend lying on her back in bed, arms spread, each hand clutched to a side of the bed to keep the bed—and herself—from flying into outer space.

She finished by saying, "That was the best weekend of my life."

After you cut the plants, you hang them for a week to dry. I can't tell you many stories about this because there are only two things you can do wrong: don't dry them enough, and they get moldy; or dry them too much, and they get crispy. I've made both of those mistakes more than once. It only took me a couple of years to figure out that I should run a dehumidifier in the wet winter, and not in the dry summer.

Then you cure the plants. Proper curing is important because it prevents buds from molding and improves their potency, smell, and taste. As I mentioned, plants don't die immediately when you cut them down, and in marijuana, under specific conditions various nonpsychoactive chemicals can continue for some time to turn into THC. Proper curing can also prevent the evaporation of some aromatic compounds that give marijuana the smells so beloved of so many stoners—that "warm smell of colitas," as The Eagles put it, "rising up through the air." And it provides the right conditions for enzymes to break down sugars produced as chlorophyll decomposes, sugars that can lend a harsh taste to the smoke.

The key is to provide those conditions

I start by cutting branches, buds attached, into lengths I can fit into paper bags—one bag per plant, pharmacy bags for tiny plants, lunch bags for smallish plants, and multiple bags for big ones.

After that, the process becomes remarkably complicated and delicate. It's hard to say whether it's more of a science or an art form. Entire chapters in books have been devoted to discussions of the process, and I've seen growers nearly come to blows defending their recipes. Some recipes involve sealing buds in containers, then intermittently "burping" the containers to allow in new air. Some argue for the use of humidity packs. Some blasphemers suggest using ovens or even microwaves. Other people respond by suggesting these blasphemers be burned at the stake on a fire made of well-dried marijuana stems.

Some people spend years of trial and error to find the best way.

Or you can do it my way.

A few years ago, a friend visited from Arizona. At one point we were sitting in my living room. He mentioned, "Your bud is always exquisitely cured. What's your secret?"

I pointed across the room to a pile of filled paper bags on the floor. I said, "After I bag them, I leave them there until I hear from the trimmer that she's ready for some more work, then I take them to her place."

The key to exquisite curing, I've learned, is to live where the temperature and humidity happen to be perfect.

If I lived anywhere else, I'd probably mess it up.

Trimmers can mess up perfect cures, too. I've gotten back trimmed bud that had a terrible cat-piss ammonia smell. That smell comes from mold. I presume the trimmer stored the bud in a working rice steamer kept in the wettest corner of a damp basement. I've also gotten back bud dry enough that if you touch it, it crumbles. I presume the trimmer stored these on the pad of a wood stove, then popped them into a sealed jar with a bunch of silica gel packets. I tried rehydrating them, following true and real recipes I found on the internet. These led to crumbly bud that had a terrible cat-piss ammonia smell.

Moral of the story: find different trimmers.

*

And sometimes trimmers steal. Just today I fired a trimmer for stealing. I'd noticed that the pot I got back from him was light and lacked big buds. Then—and this sort of craziness seems to characterize pot-world, and now that I think about it, human interactions in general—I almost simultaneously received a note from the trimmer and one from some unknown friend of his: The trimmer's note said his cousin had visited from Sacramento and high-graded my pot, that is, stolen all the big buds. The second note said, "I love [the trimmer] like a brother, but he destroys every situation he gets into, in this case by stealing. I'm honest, however, and if you'd like to buy pot from me, here's what I have available."

Despite the thefts, I had to laugh. I'll avoid the whole lot of them, thanks. And of course it was immediately clear to me that on learning his friend was going to rat him out, the trimmer had invented a "cousin from Sacramento" to preserve some dignity.

Stoners gonna stoner.

Such is life in pot-world.

Such is life, it seems, among humans.

And for all I know such is life among penguins, pandas, and porpoises.

When Tim and Mario started teaching me to grow, I marveled at their ability to identify strains at a glance. It was magic! To me the plants all just looked like marijuana. And to adapt Ronald Reagan's famous saying about redwood trees: if you've seen one marijuana plant, you've seen them all.

But while I've always known Ronald Reagan was wrong, I soon learned how wrong I was as well. In a few months I could identify one strain, and then another, and another.

Some growers specialize in one strain, growing only that plant for decades. I respect that devotion, as with each grow the human gets to better know the needs of the plant. Other growers—both Tim and Mario fall into this category—grow one strain at a time but often switch between grows. This makes a lot of sense, as it allows your care to be standardized across your grow. Trainwreck, for example, is a heavy feeder, while Dr. Grinspoon burns if you even say the words "ammonium nitrate" in hearing distance. Growing multiple strains at once means you need to pay individual attention to each plant, which, rewarding as that may be, can be a pain in the ass if you have a hundred or more plants.

And of course there are lots of growers who couldn't care less what strains they grow, so long as the end result is more green for their pockets.

I'm not so much like any of those. I love falling in love with each new strain. I love learning that the scent of Cinderella99 is a delicious and delicate swirl of lemon, orange, cinnamon, and pine, and I love learning—though this makes things harder—that she's difficult to clone. I love learning that the leaves of Pineapple Express are long and slender, while those of Grandmother Purple are short and wide. I love how different strains smell different, even when not in bloom, and I love learning the textures and tastes of those smells. I love the purple tint of the stems of Trainwreck, and I love the white-as-snow immature stigmata of Jamaican Dream. I loved that, spontaneously for about a year, immature stigmata of C4 were neon blue, and I loved hoping that color would last till harvest. I loved learning that it didn't, and to this day I love neither knowing what made them turn that color nor what eventually made them stop. I love learning which strains are susceptible to mites, mold, mildew, or scale—and which are not.

I love poring over websites selling seeds, making lists of strains I'd love to try, checking those lists twice, tossing the lists and starting over, and finally getting new seeds. I love trading strains with friends—imagining the lives the plants will have in their new homes and giving a good home to the plants I receive in return.

I grow probably fifteen or twenty strains. Sometimes I get new ones. Sometimes old ones drift away.

I can tell the difference in strains now at a glance, or a smell, or a touch. I love that.

*

The other day Tim let me know he was coming for a visit.

I said, "Great! You want to bring me a few new strains?"

He started laughing, said, "Thank God you're interested in growing plants instead of raising children, or you'd be living a remake of that old Myrna Loy flick *Cheaper by the Dozen*."

"Come on," I said. "Just a couple."

"I am not," he responded, still laughing, "going to enable your obsession with diversity."

Identifying a strain, though, can be elusive, like identifying a smell. Is that really a swirl of lemon, orange, cinnamon, and pine—or is it something else? Did I just, out of nowhere, get a whiff of the cinnamon rolls my mother used to make?

In other words, although I say I can tell at a glance the difference between strains, I still put tags in the pots to identify them. At first— I'm not sure why, but I think it's because I do everything wrong at first—I'd write numbers on tags, and on a piece of paper I'd write that the number one equals Trainwreck, number two equals Afwreck, and so on. It only took me a couple of years to figure out I didn't need the paper; I could just write TW or AF on the tag itself. I usually get there in the end.

But sometimes when I make clones I mess up and write the wrong strain on the tag, or sometimes during transplanting I lose a tag and have to rely on my ability to tell the strains apart.

Which, it ends up, is not quite as good as I sometimes like to believe.

This isn't a problem when the tag gets lost during the bloom phase, since the buds are nearly always easy to differentiate. Blood Orange smells remarkably like its name, as does Blueberry Kush. Double Black smells like cat piss but different than the cat-piss smell that comes from mold, and some of the kushes smell like baby shit. You'll note I don't grow those particular kushes.

The problem comes when the tag is lost when the plant is in veg. If you recall, clones are the same age as the plant from whom—I know we're supposed to say "which" but the plants are individuals—you take a cutting, so you need to take clones before moving the plants from veg to bloom. This means a mistake here can easily replicate through generations.

Sometimes I end up with a plant marked Jamaican Dream that definitely has Thai buds.

Which means I have a whole new generation of Thai marked JD.

I understand why Tim and Mario grow only one strain at a time.

But I'm nothing if not stubborn—as well as obsessed with diversity—so I keep growing a bunch of strains while devising increasingly Byzantine tag marking schemes—sometimes involving filling notebook after notebook with translations of the damn marks—to track and eventually identify the plants in question. I'll spare you the details of these unnecessarily complicated schemes and just say that, evidently, I'm as obsessed with bizarre tracking systems as I am with diversity of strains.

Someday, if you ask nicely, I'll show you the notebooks.

Another problem is what to do with your stems. As with leaves, some people, especially in cities, bag them and toss the bags into dumpsters. People in the country can burn them in their woodstoves, a plan that doesn't work quite so well for urban or suburban stealth grows, since the smoke smells like you're trying to replicate Woodstock in your living room. The stems can be big enough for composting to be slow and to require a sizeable compost heap.

Since I'm normally the only person who walks down the path from my mom's house to mine, for a few months, when I started, I lined the stems along the path, so I could watch the process of these stems becoming part of the forest. It was fun to watch fungi colonize them, then watch banana slugs eat the fungi and carry nutrients from the stems to feed different parts of the forest.

I quickly realized, however, that if any teenagers happened to be walking through the forest, leaving marijuana stems along the path would be like handing them a treasure map. So I gathered the long row of stems and scattered them throughout the forest. That's what I've done with all stems since. It still makes me happy when I wander off the path, to see the remains of old stems, whitened by fungi and slugs and who knows whom else, slowly mixing with duff, becoming part of the redwood trees, part of the forest.

After the buds are cured, they're trimmed: shaped and smoothed by cutting away small leaves—called sugar leaves—amidst the flowers.

There's a part of me that doesn't understand the point of trimming. The sugar leaves are themselves covered with trichomes, so you're removing lots of perfectly good trichomes for primarily cosmetic reasons.

On the other hand, well-trimmed buds sure do look real purdy.

I shouldn't be so glib, because trimming can be described as a form of meditation, an act of holy consecration and worship, a way to see the divine made manifest in the world, to see the green goddess in the buds. Repetition has long been known as one way to experience ecstatic trance: chanting, drumming, dancing, spinning, using prayer beads, prostrations. And trimming is nothing if not repetitious.

You pick up a short length of branch by its lower end. You use your left hand, because trimming scissors are right-handed, which means lefties as always suffer mainly in silence against the oppressiveness of the master hand. Those of us in this most oppressed of all categories are required by this dextro-supremacist culture to use the master's tools to trim the master's—or anyone else's—buds.

Think on that, and if you're right-handed, check your privilege, buster, because some day the revolution will come, and when it does. . . Well, let's just say they don't call us lefties *sinister* for nothing.

I guess I drifted away from the spiritual vibe of trimming. If I just focus on the repetition, the feelings of anger and resentment will fade.

Small buds grow from the sides of the branches, a couple of inches apart. Small sugar leaves grow from the bases of these buds and curl around them. Cut these. Also cut any leaves poking out from the buds. Then cut the bud from the branch, and put it on a tray. Make your way up the branch. When you've trimmed all the buds from one branch, put the branch aside and pick up another.

Save all those removed sugar leaves—called trim—in another pile. Add the really tiny buds—called popcorn—to this pile. We'll return to that pile later.

The stems at the tops of the plants yield the colas, those collections of buds that will be anywhere from the size of a Christmas tree light up to a baseball bat—these latter sometimes called, and don't blame me for the vulgarity, donkey dongs. These colas aren't one large bud but rather masses of smaller buds. It can happen—and of course I've done this more times than I can count—that removing sugar leaves from these colas reveals gaps between the various buds. Gaps are aesthetically unpleasing, so when that happens you have to cut that small bud below the gap away from the cola. This may reveal yet another gap, which means you have to cut the next bud and the next, until before you know it you've reduced your donkey dong down to a collection of buds the size of superballs.

Then you pick up the next branch, and start the process over. You do this for days, or until you've finished all the branches and stems, or until you achieve enlightenment through this meditative repetition.

Or until you get fed up and hire someone else to trim.

Perceiving trimming as meditation is only one perspective. Another is represented by the bumper sticker I've not infrequently seen in this town—remember, this is marijuana country—announcing simply, TRIMMING SUCKS.

I tend to fall into the latter camp.

I used to trim my own bud. Trimmers can, I think, be put into four broad categories: slow and sloppy, fast and sloppy, slow and meticulous, and fast and meticulous. Let's leave off the first two categories, since sloppy trimming doesn't help cosmetically, which is, if you recall, the primary point of trimming. I've seen trimmers who cut off a few of the pokiest leaves and didn't even bother to cut the buds from the stems. Not surprisingly, these trimmers never got paid. I'm in the slow and meticulous category, which could be one reason I'm also in the "trimming sucks" category.

Here's my prototypical trimming experience. I grab a bunch of paper bags full of cured buds on branches and go to my mom's house.

She complains about the smell. We put on an episode of *Poirot*. I sit on the floor with a tray in front of me to catch the trim, pull out a branch, grab the scissors and start. David Suchet and Hugh Fraser are perfect as Poirot and Hastings. My mom complains about the smell. I complete one bud, then another, then another. My mom complains about the smell. After an hour, I'm delighted with my progress, and decide to weigh the trimmed buds and see how I'm doing. They total about seven grams, or a little under a quarter of an ounce.

I do the math. At the time the going rate for trimming was $200/lb. That converts to $12.50/ounce. By trimming it myself instead of paying someone, I was saving myself about $3.12/hour. Admittedly I was watching *Poirot* with my mom, so how bad could it be? But honestly, I made more than that per hour working at a Round the Corner burger joint in high school in 1979.

If I'm going to meditate, I think I'll just take long walks through the forest and hand off the trimming to someone else.

Many people wear latex gloves when trimming, because otherwise your fingers get sticky from the THC that rubs off as you handle the buds. Other people don't, however, preferring to let their hands get dark and sticky, then to roll this sticky film into balls that can be smoked or sold. These are called finger hash, and are considered by some to be among the highest quality hash.

Which brings us to trim and popcorn. You can compost this or throw it away, but you can also sell it for $25 to $150 per pound. Or you can smoke it; it gets the job done, and buds sell for twelve to twenty-five times the price of trim. While trim might be weaker—so smoke a little more—popcorn buds are still buds, albeit scrawny. Most people grind their bud before smoking it, so size doesn't matter. Like the shoemaker who wears leftovers because her best work goes to market, a lot of growers smoke trim.

If you're not going to compost, sell, or smoke it, the question becomes: How can you separate THC from trim? There are four common methods. The oldest is to physically knock off trichomes. People have been doing this for as long as they've been smoking marijuana, for example putting trim or buds into a woven basket covered by a cloth, inverting the basket, and tapping on the cloth. This shakes off trichomes. They fall through the cloth.

You can also buy a tumbler online to knock them off automatically. It's a hollow cylinder surrounded by fine screen, attached lengthwise to a horizontal rod inside a tub. You put trim and some superballs into the cylinder, then turn on an electric motor that rotates the cylinder at twenty revolutions per minute. Wooden ribs inside the cylinder force the contents to tumble instead of slide. The tumbling and the smacking by superballs knocks off trichomes, which fall to the bottom as a barely sticky powder called kief, or kief hash.

These machines cost from $500 to $1,000, and consist of a ten-dollar tote, a twenty-dollar electric motor, a five-dollar cord and switch, a two-dollar rod, and a fifteen-dollar cylinder. They don't even supply superballs (144 for fifteen seventy-five; you only need three, but for this price how can you refuse?). Assembly takes less than thirty minutes.

The primary winners in gold rushes aren't usually the miners but rather their suppliers.

After a few runs, collect kief from the tub bottom. Pro-tip: if you have pets, cover the tub, or their hair will end up inside. Trichomes stick to hair—not a good aesthetic, and you know what burning hair smells like.

A second way of separating trichomes from leaves consists of putting frozen trim into ice water, then using a cake beater to knock off the trichomes. Then filter the slurry through a series of increasingly fine meshes. Put aside the wet trim to compost. Scrape off the pasty residue, called bubble hash, from each of the meshes. The finer the mesh, the better quality the hash.

You can also use trim for cooking. Because THC is an oil, it binds to fat. Put trim and butter in a pot, turn on the heat, and let this go a couple of hours, stirring occasionally. Don't do this at your mother's house, or for the next month she'll quite rightly complain about the smell, something like overcooked brassica and generalized skunk. Strain this mess through a cheesecloth into another pot. Let sit till butter congeals. Use butter to cook brownies, cookies, and so on. Give them to friends, who will then sit motionless on the couch through several episodes of the original *Star Trek*.

Since I live in a forest, oftentimes people give me their stems, leaves, or spent trim from kief or bubble hash to dispose of. I'm glad to do it, since the forest is hungry.

But disposal of spent trim from making butter always brings me a moral dilemma. I don't want to throw it away or burn it in the fireplace because the trim is infused with butter, a high quality, high calorie food that would be snapped up by all sorts of animals, from bears to slugs; and on the other hand I don't want to throw it in the forest because the butter is infused with THC and might get these creatures stoned.

A veterinarian told me she often receives frantic calls from people whose dogs are lethargic, barely willing to stand, eyes unfocused. The vet always asks if there's pot in the house. Dogs love butter, and they also often love to eat buds. Dogs don't die of it, and in a few cases the dogs evidently like feeling stoned enough that they seek it out time after time.

But I don't want to be responsible for couch-locked bears, or especially small animals who might get eaten. Although if slugs ate it, I'm not sure how we'd tell if they were stoned.

On a side note, banana slugs are known for sex that lasts twenty-four hours at a time, and who knows how long that would be in marijuana-fractured seconds?

I haven't resolved this dilemma. I've thought about breaking the butter balls into pieces and throwing them into the ocean, but I'm not convinced it wouldn't couch-lock fish. There *has* been one study on whether THC affects fish, but it was done on factory farmed fish crammed fin-by-gill to see if it would slightly alleviate their terror and panic (instead of, I don't know, raising them in a way that isn't a form of hell on earth). Not surprisingly, the fish were no less terrorized. And I don't want to imagine what marijuana-fractured seconds, paranoia, and hallucinations might have felt like for them under those conditions. Honestly, I kind of hope some fish capture the people who did this and put them through that same sort of hell.

Shoot, I need to readjust my attitude again. Maybe I need to do some more trimming.

The final common way to separate trichomes from trim involves butane. Yes, *that* butane, the flammable one. The one that causes explosions. Combine butane and stoners, and imagine the possibilities. The Eureka Fire Department doesn't have to imagine them, since this extraction is a primary cause of house fires in Humboldt County.

You put your trim in some sort of cylinder, flush butane through it, and the butane bonds with THC and other cannabinoids. Then you evaporate the butane, and you've got what's called shatter—because it forms brittle, sticky sheets that shatter when bent—with THC concentrations up to 90 percent.

The cylinder can be as simple as a Pringles can with a hole in the bottom. In this case the butane escapes into the room. Then maybe your friend comes in smoking a joint. Then whoever remains calls the fire department. I've seen more than my share of growers with scarred arms from doing this.

Making shatter can also be more complicated and expensive. When researching this book, I spoke with someone who has been designing and making butane extractors since the seventies. Now he runs a company manufacturing them to sell to aboveground marijuana businesses. I asked him how much his extractors cost.

He said, "We have one under six figures—a stripped down model that sells for $35,000—but most run two to three hundred thousand."

The cheapest extractors I've seen online still cost several thousand dollars.

I see why so many people choose Pringles cans.

Interlude

On a dark desert highway
Cool wind in my hair
Warm smell of colitas
Rising up through the air
Up ahead in the distance
I saw a shimmering light
I sparked one up, it kicked right in
I had to stop for a bite

Then I stood in the doorway
Of a Taco Bell
And I was thinking to myself
This could be Heaven or more likely Hell
Then I lit up a fatty
And it blew me away
There were voices down the corridor
I thought I heard them say

Welcome to the buds from California
Such a lovely taste (such a lovely taste)
But they'll grow your waist
You'll need plenty of food with the buds from California
Any time of year (any time of year)
A toke will bring you cheer

My tastes have definitely shifted
I do love those bacon ends.
And lots of pretty, pretty joys
Called m&ms
How they dance on those tastebuds
Sweet sugar mess
Some eat and remember
I eat and forget

So I called up the doctor
Said please tuck my behind
I haven't had a small rear end
Since I was twenty-nine
But still those doughnuts keep calling from far away
Wake me up in the middle of the night
Just to hear them say
Welcome to those buds from California
Welcome to the buds from California
Such a nice surprise (such a nice surprise)
I'm smokin' it up with the buds from California
It's a nice surprise, but now I've got big thighs

Cupcakes every evening
Sweet Italian ice
And I say, "We are all just prisoners here, of Mister Nice."

And in my gastric chamber
Food stagnates from my feast
But when I've got the munchies
I don't care in the least

Last thing I remember, I was
Reaching for a s'more
I had to find a diet plan back
To the weight I was before

Relax, said the fat cells
We are programmed to receive
You can diet any time you'd like
But we will never leave

CHAPTER 5

Pests

I know someone who had $100,000 in cash almost stolen by bears.
She'd been growing and distributing for a few years and faced the same problem a lot of people associated with marijuana do, which is where to put the cash. You can't just deposit it in a bank, since if you deposit $10,000 at once, or even smaller amounts in a way someone at the bank deems suspicious, banks are required to report the activity to the federal government. And they do. In just one year, banks filed more than 700,000 suspicious activity reports. There are more than a hundred multi-agency task forces that comb through bank records, looking for money the feds can seize, even when there's not even an accusation of illegal activity. The feds have seized money deposited by dairy farmers, a cash-only restaurant, a family-run candy and cigarette distributor, an army sergeant saving money for his daughters' college funds (cash, because he didn't trust banks through the 2008 banking crisis so kept cash in his basement to deposit after the crisis was over), and so many others.[1]

Putting the money in your checking account is out.

So are safe deposit boxes, in part because safe deposit boxes are too small to hold much cash, and in part because if the feds go after your grow, they can also get a search warrant for your box, and steal—sorry, seize—your cash to use as evidence of illegal activities.

It can also be problematic to buy real estate unless you can show how you got the money or might have gotten the money, or can pretend

---

[1] Shaila Dawan, "Law Lets I.R.S. Seize Accounts on Suspicion, No Crime Required," *New York Times*, October 25, 2014, accessed October 31, 2019, https://www.nytimes.com/2014/10/26/us/law-lets-irs-seize-accounts-on-suspicion-no-crime-required.html.

that you got the money. Some people are kind of stupid this way. I read about one guy in his twenties who got arrested after he purchased his third home with cash without having any remotely reasonable way of showing income. He also had two new BMWs and a new SUV.

I spoke with one grower who said, "A popular method for payment around my neck of the redwoods is blank money orders. People send blank ones from the East, and then the receiver uses them to pay bills. It's essentially a thousand-dollar bill, although one of my ex-boyfriends cashed too many, and the IRS wanted to know where they came from. He's on the run now, and of all the guys I've met in the Emerald Triangle, he deserves it most. So as much as I hate to say it, score one for the IRS."

Keeping the money in your house is generally out, too, because, to be honest, people suck. Or more accurately, a lot of individuals are nice, but people in general suck. Or no, that's not true. What is true is that some people suck, and the larger the population, the greater the chance there'll be individuals, maybe a lot of them, who suck. There are, for example, a lot of people out there who, if they knew you had $100,000 in cash in your home, would without hesitation kill you and take it. Hell, there are a lot who would kill you for a lot less. Double hell, there are people on death row who killed over $5, $10, five pain pills, $25, $100—you name it.

I'm not necessarily talking about your friends, although just today I heard about someone in this town who shot a man and his wife, with whom he had evidently until that night been friends, because of a dispute over the price of firewood. The victims lived, but I'm presuming the friendship didn't.

I once read an interview with a high-stakes poker player who mentioned having to carefully vet whoever cleaned his home, because his livelihood required him to often have scores of thousands in cash on hand. He said he'd have to be able to trust his housekeeper to lift a tall stack of hundred dollar bills to clean the table under it, then put it back exactly as it was and not tell too many friends about having done that.

I've been around friends and acquaintances with stacks of money and it never occurred to me to take any of it; that's kind of the point of friendship, isn't it? It's also, of course, kind of the point of being a decent person. If the money belonged to ExxonMobil and not a human being, we might have a different discussion.

The problem comes at the level of friends of friends, and then the friends of those friends, and then their friends, and on out. Let's say you have $100,000 in cash at your house. Your friends are decent people, so you're not worried about them. So you let slip to a friend that you have this money at your house, and then this friend lets slip to his friend, who lets slip to her friend, who lets slip to his friend—who gets some bright ideas.

This happens all the time.

A couple of examples. Long before I started growing, my mom had a non-marijuana flower garden that she loved. She grew too old to weed it by herself. Her good-for-nothing son—that would be me, and it's my words, not hers—was not fond of weeding and preferred paying some teenager to help. Not knowing any teenagers ourselves, we asked a neighbor. That neighbor knew a family who needed some money. We hired their fourteen-year-old son to come over every Saturday for a few hours. One Saturday I had an event in Eugene, Oregon, about four hours north of here. I thought it would be a nice ride for my mom, so she told the teen we'd be gone that day. He told his older brother, who told his friend, and when my mom and I got home from the event, the house had been cleaned out and my truck had been stolen, used to transport their haul. The thieves even stole hand-sewn quilts that took my mom a year each to make.

Depending on how you count it, that's only three or four degrees of separation from my mom.

Addendum to this story: the primary thief got caught and sent down for fifty-four months, and when he got out he was caught again within a month, this time with $120,000 worth of stolen items, including several handguns. He went down for seven years for that one, got out, and within months was caught again and sent away on three strikes.

Second addendum to that story: my mom had a few gold coins the guy didn't find. She kept them at the bottom of a little basket of dried lavender. Had he picked it up, he would have found it weighed far too much for dried flowers. But he didn't pick it up. Too bad, so sad.

Another example. The couple who just got shot are acquaintances of a friend of mine. If I had money here—and for the record, I don't keep anything beyond petty cash at my house, or anywhere else for that matter—I would trust my friend to know about it. Would I trust his acquaintances? Hell, no. Would I trust their friend who shot them? Sure, but only to murder me and steal everything I have. I learned tonight from my friend that the shooter is a twice-convicted violent felon, and the victims in this case have refused to tell the police his name because they know that if they do, he'll come back and kill them. My friend was visibly uncomfortable talking about the guy even just to me, without using the guy's name. And my friend is no stranger to violence and danger himself. He has spent time in prison. And a couple of months ago, in the midst of an MRI he started complaining about pain in his back. It ends up that for the past thirty years he's had a steel-jacketed bullet lodged near his spine. "I guess I must have forgotten about that particular time I got shot," he told me. And *he* is scared to talk about the guy. That's the sort of guy the shooter is.

And that's only three degrees of separation from me.

So you can't keep cash at your house.

My friend who was looking for a place to rest her cash knew someone who owned 180 acres of second-growth, mixed redwood/cedar forest. The guy is also a grower, and he bought the land to protect it. The land is rough terrain, much of it steep, much of it covered in dense huckleberry/salal undergrowth. To get to the path that leads to his home you have to drive a rutted road, park, and then ford a knee-deep rocky stream. He and his family are the only ones who ever walk on the land, and they mainly stay on the paths. He said my friend could hide the money somewhere—he wouldn't know where, so even though she trusted him, she didn't have to—and could come get it whenever she wanted.

She vacuum-sealed the cash—a combo of hundreds, fifties, and twenties that took up a large USPS flat-rate priority box, about twelve by twelve by six inches—and put that inside a black garbage bag, which she tightly wrapped and then excessively taped, although I'm not sure it's possible to excessively tape a bag holding your life savings. She took it to the guy's land, set off on a path, and when it felt right took one game trail, then another, then another, and finally started crawling through underbrush till she found a downed tree beneath which some creature had dug, then abandoned, a small den. She crawled in, pushed the bundle to the back, crawled out.

She memorized the area, took copious notes and even more copious digital photographs all the way to the trail—honestly, I can imagine doing this and not being able to find my way back—and then went home, pleased with having found such a safe solution to the problem of what to do with her cash, and thankful to the friend for enabling it.

But neither of them counted on bears.

Six months later she needed some cash and returned to the land. She parked, waded, walked, stopped and said hello to her friend, walked some more, walked more after that, and then crawled. As she crawled, she realized a mistake she'd made. She should have packed the cash in ten bundles of 10K each instead of one big bundle, so she could have just grabbed a bundle and left. This way she had to take the whole bundle home, seal it up again—they don't as of yet make battery-powered vacuum sealers, and thanks be to Humbaba and other forest deities as well as the grower who bought the land that there were no electrical outlets in the forest—and bring it back out. But then again, she was getting up close and personal with a beautiful forest, and how bad can that be?

She got to her cache, and something was very wrong. The forest floor was covered in cash. She panicked. This was her life savings, stolen. How did someone find her hiding place? Never for a moment did she think her friend stole it, but who did?

Then it occurred to her that if some thief had found her cash, he wouldn't have left any behind. She started scooping up the wet, muddy money and putting it in the plastic bag she'd brought to carry home her cash.

On the way out she thought about it, and realized: *bears*. They'd found her bag, and being bears, wondered what it was. They'd opened it, tossed it around, smelled it, chewed on it a little, and when they realized it wasn't edible had walked away.

She was glad we don't use fish as currency.

She would have laughed, but she hadn't yet counted the money.

She took it home, put plastic over her bed—the money was muddy, after all—and dried it. But the suspense was killing her, and she started counting it wet. Twenty, forty, sixty, eighty, one. Twenty, forty, sixty, eighty, two.

It was all there. Every dollar.

She had no idea how long after she'd left it that the bears had gotten into her money, but presumably the cash had been out for weeks or months. She was glad this region has thick undergrowth. She'd routinely stood in forests experiencing gale force winds at the tops of trees, with not a whisper at ground level, such is the windbreaking power of tall trees and thick underbrush.

She was glad she hadn't hidden the money in a desert, or it would have blown away like the gold dust at the end of *The Treasure of the Sierra Madre*. And she didn't think she would have been able to laugh about it.

Storing one's money in a forest is common enough to have a name: "I'm going to go make a deposit in the bank of the woods."

She was a first-generation American. Her grandparents were from eastern Poland and survived the Soviet invasion and occupation by keeping their heads down, then survived the Nazi invasion and occupation the same way. Her mother was born in early 1944, just in time to be carried by her parents to the West, where they ended up in a displaced persons camp. A few years later they were accepted into the United States.

Her grandparents worked hard but were solidly lower-middle class. Her parents met in the early sixties, had a few kids, and remained lower-middle class.

When my friend had her money spread all over her bed, she thought very seriously about taking a picture of it and sending it to her parents. She even thought about including the caption, "Made it, Ma! Top of the world!" She didn't, though, not only because saying that didn't end well for Cagney; but mainly because her parents had no idea she was growing pot. She'd always told them she made her living growing heirloom organic garlic for a gourmet market, and while she was never sure whether or not they believed her, she suspected a picture of her sitting on her bed with $100,000 in literally dirty money would not have pushed the belief needle in the right direction.

Another grower had just sold several pounds and had eight thousand in cash in a bag on the console of her crew cab truck. She told me, "After making the drop I picked up a couple of friends at the airport. They wanted to see the harbor, so we drove on down. My two dogs were with me. As we're rolling to a stop one dog got it into her head to jump out the back window. I stopped the car and took off after her. But I was too freaked out to remember to put it in park. Of course the truck started rolling. Right toward the harbor. My friend in the front seat had my other dog, who weighs eighty pounds, on her lap, so she had to steer the wheel with her left hand and try to push the dog off her lap with her right. She got him on the floor and kicked/crawled her way into the driver's seat. But as she did this, she kicked my bag full of cash out the open door. I caught my dog and looked around to see my truck rolling toward the harbor and hundreds of twenty-dollar bills floating through the air like it was some sort of game show.

"Fortunately, my friend stopped the car before it went into the drink, and we got all the money back, but it was one of those moments where I thought, 'What has happened to my life?'

"Oh, and some cops pulled into the parking lot soon after, but thank the goddess we'd gotten all the cash collected by then."

*

Napoleon famously commented that an army marches on its stomach. Many in marijuana culture have commented—though not so famously, and often anonymously—that marijuana wholesaling, transportation, and distribution relies on turkey bags, ziplock bags, and meal sealers.

Someone who has been wholesaling marijuana for the last fifteen years told me, "Without turkey bags this business wouldn't be possible. This is the first place I've lived where the local paper has ads in September and October saying, 'Turkey bags are on sale for harvest time.' Who puts out ads for turkey bags? And there are billboards for turkey bags!"

"Why turkey bags?"

"They hold a pound of marijuana very nicely, and cut down on odors."

I asked her about ziplock bags.

She said, "I swear, the people at the grocery store must think I have fifteen children, with the number of ziplock bags I go through. Except of course this is marijuana country, so everyone knows what they're for." She paused, then said, "What's really made this industry possible, though, are meal-sealers. Two layers of double-vacuum seal and there are no odors, so it can be mailed or muled with no telltale scent. I'm not a particularly big wholesaler, but I go through a sealer every six months. At one point I bought an industrial sealer, and it lasted a couple of years, but when it crapped out, I couldn't fix it, so it ended up being more economical to buy cheap ones and consider them disposable."

I asked, "How did you get started?"

"I was living in the Midwest and was tired of being poor. So I moved to the Emerald Triangle and tried to figure out how to make marijuana work. The American Dream, you know?"

"Did you have contacts for pot when you moved out here?"

"I had one. He was a small grower whose wholesaler went out of business because his primary mule got arrested transporting pot through South Dakota. He had some pot that needed moving, and I had no cash, so he gave it to me on consignment. I was soon able to pay him back and buy more of his pot. But I had to develop more contacts, because this grower wasn't enough to supply demand."

"How did you find those contacts? You can't look in the Yellow Pages."

"You can actually look on Craigslist. But mostly I just asked people point-blank. If they didn't grow, they had a cousin who did."

"And how did you know whom to trust?"

"You don't. You can't. There's no way to know. It's scary, because you could end up with all sorts of strange people showing up at your house thinking you have cash. That's part of the downside: the potential for home invasion. If people think you're involved, they may assume you've got lots of cash lying around. Or at least it's worth their while to find out. So that's the risk. And you don't want all these people up in your business."

I thought about someone I'd heard of who got tired of having cash stolen from his home, so he installed a big safe in his floor. One day when he was gone, thieves used a jackhammer to rip the safe from the floor and take it with them. After that he took to staying home all the time holding a gun and smoking pot. That didn't work either as thieves came back with bigger guns and ripped him off again. And again. After that he went a bit crazy, insisting to any of his friends who still came to visit that people were in his attic, waiting for him to fall asleep so they could rob him. One day he ran into the street with his gun and started shooting at phantoms inside his house. Last I heard, his sister came from Wisconsin to take him home.

The woman continued, "Of course, the alternative is to go to them, which can be just as scary. Especially as a woman. I've met growers in state parks, I've met them at specific turnouts on the sides of highways, I've been to their houses. It's also how I've ended up with $40,000 in a knapsack in a motel parking lot in the pitch dark, waiting for someone I've never met to bring me a garbage bag full of marijuana. I stood there thinking, 'How did this happen to my life? Will I still be alive tomorrow? It's like something from a bad movie.' But it all went fine."

"Have you ever been ripped off?"

She laughed, somewhere between bitterly and maniacally. "All the time. You have to include it as a cost of doing business, because you can't go to court. I know some men who, when this happens, round up their buddies and go take care of it."

I said, "I was just talking to someone growing on land without permission of the absentee landowner, right near a meth-addict encampment. I asked how he keeps them from stealing his pot, and he responded, 'You pay close attention, and the first one who does it you beat the shit out of him—and I mean beat him good—and then tell him to tell all his friends to keep out. Works great.'"

She said, "There's definitely violence in this culture. But that's not an option for me. Sure, I've got big friends who would not only be willing but eager to do that for me—shall we talk about Jimmy the Impaler? But I personally find that immoral. I got into this business in part because marijuana makes people feel good, and I don't want to inflict violence on anyone. Consequently, I've been ripped off perhaps more than some. An option I have strongly considered, especially for outdoor growers, is to sneak in a bunch of male plants near their grow."

She continued, "This business is not all elves and strawberries. But I also have made a lot of money. The people who've ripped me off are just being stupid. We could have made a lot more money working together long-term: there are people I've been working with for more than a decade now, and we go to each other's children's weddings. There are people who will with no problem front me twenty pounds of marijuana because they know I'm good for it. And likewise, just before harvest, if I'm flush and they're in trouble, I'll front them the cash."

I asked, "How do you get ripped off? Do they pull out a gun?"

"That's happened to people I know, but never to me. Mainly with me they've given me short pounds, or there are a lot of seeds, or the marijuana is just crap and the buyers don't like it. That's not always a rip-off. Sometimes it's a mistake, and they give me more pot to make up for it. And sometimes it *is* a rip-off, because they say they'll make it right but they never show up, and it becomes quite clear they've got crap product and they know it.

"Oh, here's a great example," she said. "On the recommendation of a friend I paid cash up front for ten pounds. But the grower didn't show up at the drop to deliver the marijuana. And then I found out he'd sold a thousand pounds when he only had a hundred to sell. He did this, I later discovered, because he's a heroin addict. So he was shooting up all of our money, and people were pissed.

"I knew where his grow was, so I went up there. He hadn't been there for weeks. His business partners were understandably freaked out—they were having irate buyers show up all hours of day and night, many of whom did not have my scruples. It's not uncommon in those situations for the people who've been ripped off to say, 'Nice TV. It's mine now. So's your truck. And it doesn't matter if you give me the pink slip since I have a friend who runs a chop shop. Don't worry, I'm only going to take what's owed me, plus a 20 percent asshole surcharge.' This is common enough, and it's often called 'hill justice.' But like I said, that's not my way.

"In this case the junkie had a girlfriend half his age who'd just had a baby. So I sat her down and told her very bluntly that this was never going to get better and that she needed to get out while she was still alive. I made her tell me where her family was, and then I put her in my car and drove her to the bus station. We called her mom from the station, and I bought her a ticket back up the Coast. Her family was happy to know she would be safe and was going to help her.

"You can't hide the fact that there's a lot of exploitation in this industry, and a lot of vulnerable people who get hurt." She thought a moment, then said, "I never got my money back, but at least that girl and her baby are safe."

Not everyone in marijuana culture is safe. I don't know anyone who has been murdered because of pot. But it happens. In only one year, 2020, fourteen people were murdered just in Riverside County in Southern California associated with illegal marijuana operations, including seven people at one grow scene, where police also found 1,000 pounds of pot.

In 2019, a postal carrier was murdered by men who stole a package of marijuana she was unknowingly carrying. Also in 2019, a Louisiana marijuana dealer pled guilty to paying an associate $5,000 to kill someone who'd stolen from him. This dealer was also involved in dog fighting. Not every marijuana dealer is a nice person.

Legal marijuana dealers get killed, too. Again in 2019, a Silicon Valley entrepreneur who had diversified into marijuana production was killed by some of his employees and their friends. Why? Because he had money.

I asked her how she transports the pot after she buys it.

She said, "In my car. The first time I drove anywhere with fifteen pounds in the trunk I was freaking out the whole drive. But after all these years, honestly, I don't even think about it anymore. I've never even had any close calls."

I talked to other people who *have* had their share of close scrapes. One said, "I was driving back to California from Oregon with a shit-load of pot in the back of my pickup, in turkey bags inside those big forty-eight-quart coolers. It was the middle of the night. I got to the agricultural inspection station at the California border. Normally, even during the day they just wave you through, and at night the thing is closed. But they were stopping every car, checking in the back seats and in the trunks. I thought seriously about turning around, but there's no other way home that wouldn't involve a several-hour drive—and yeah, I know, when you're facing possible arrest a several-hour drive doesn't seem like a bad option, but we don't always make good choices, do we? So I waited in the queue. They got to me, and it ends up it was the start of some hunting season or another, and they were checking to make sure hunters bringing meat or carcasses had proper game tags. Great, right? Except what do you transport meat in? Coolers, a bunch of them. They took one look in the back, asked for my permit, and I told them these were vegetables from my garden up in Roseburg. They didn't believe me and asked if they could look. Fortunately, I had one cooler of vegetables from the garden of the guy I bought the pot from.

I got out, popped that open to show him the squash and other shit, and he waved me through."

I talked to someone else about his closest call transporting. He laughed, and said, "When I was seventeen, back in the seventies, a relative asked me to drive from Santa Cruz, California, where we both lived, down to Tucson, Arizona, to pick up some pot, then drive it back to Santa Cruz. He said he'd let me use his old Plymouth Duster, he'd pay for gas and for all the food I could eat on the way there and back, and on delivery he'd give me three hundred bucks. It was twelve or thirteen hours each way. What seventeen-year-old could refuse that?"

I thought about how excited I'd been when I was seventeen and my sister asked me to drive one of her vehicles from Grants, New Mexico, to Boulder, Colorado, as part of a move—and how, when I was nineteen, I drove that same sister from Boulder to where she was then living in Nevada, stopped for breakfast, and turned around and drove home—all for the fun of it. Nowadays I complain when I have to drive two miles to the grocery store.

He continued, "I drove down, stopping at more or less every fast food place on the way—don't ever promise to pay for all the food a seventeen-year-old can eat—and went to pick up the pot. My relative had told me to put as much as I could in the car, so I packed the trunk, packed the back seat, piled up the passenger side of the front seat. I even broke open packages—this was Mexican brickweed—and put them on the back panel and the dash. I was such an idiot. Anybody driving by could see these bricks of weed on the dash. What was I thinking? I drove straight through on the way back, I'm sure with a wave of skunk fanning out behind the car, and when I pulled in to my relative's driveway and he saw how I'd packed it he almost had a heart attack."

I talked to another person about his closest call transporting. He said, "It wasn't really a close call, but it was nerve-wracking. I was taking a U-Haul full of pot cross country, enough to have put me away for a long time. The highway was reduced to one-lane, stop-and-go traffic because of construction. And there was a state patrol officer directly behind me. For the first few miles I was freaking out, but at some point, the Serenity Prayer kicked in and I thought, 'Whatever is going to happen is going to happen.' For the rest of what seemed like a hundred miles I was remarkably calm. Of course, when the road opened up again and he pulled around me I realized I hadn't taken a deep breath the entire time."

And I talked to one more. He told me, "I'd taken much larger loads, but I was once transporting a few pounds in the saddlebags of my motorcycle when I came to a police roadblock. I didn't worry yet; I figured it was a sobriety checkpoint. Then I saw they weren't just checking drivers but also passengers. When it was my turn one of the cops got all nervous and told me to get off my bike. I did, and he started asking questions. It soon became clear the checkpoint was looking for someone who had just robbed a bank and made his getaway on a motorcycle. The robber was evidently dressed, as I was, all in leather. They started making noises about searching my saddlebags for the money. Of course there wasn't money in there, but there was enough weed to put me away. Finally, I heard one cop double-check something on his radio and then say, 'It's not him. Our perp is five foot eight.' I've never been so glad I'm six and a half feet tall."

I asked the woman from the Midwest, "How did you find people to buy the pot?"

She said, "The same way I found growers: I asked everyone I knew. Most said no; a few wanted to buy individual amounts, just for themselves, but I really needed to find small dealers who wanted good product. Luckily—and I swear this is not an infomercial—Humboldt County produces the best marijuana in the world. So eventually I was able to find people in the Midwest who were already dealers or who wanted to get started because they could see the amount of money to be made."

"Again, how do you know whom to trust?"

"You don't. It's a risk, and there definitely have been people who were weirded out that I asked. Some used it as an opportunity to launch into a rant about how much they hate marijuana: oops, bad vetting on my part. But worse are the ones who end up being not trustworthy. You can lose thousands of dollars."

"How do you send the pot?"

"I mail it through the post office. Everything is double vacuum sealed, then put in mylar, and then in a double-walled cardboard box."

I said, drily, "I presume you use your own return address."

She laughed. "Not quite. I use fake address labels. Something realistic. You wouldn't believe some of the stupid names people have used for their return address."

"I would believe it. I was asking the clerks at the post office, and they've told me stories of people coming in reeking of pot trying to mail packages with return addresses of 'Fred Flint Stoned,' 'I.M. High,' 'Hugh Kant Catchme,' or 'Bud Weed,' although that last one might have been real. Bad news for him since they called the cops anyway."

When you think about people moving marijuana across the country, it's pretty easy to think they used to mule it physically, in cars or trucks, but more recently they've switched to using delivery services like the postal service or UPS. But that's not accurate for a couple of reasons.

The first is that a lot of people still move it physically. I've talked to growers and wholesalers who meet up every month or two with people from Chicago or Detroit or Atlanta who are looking to score hundreds of pounds of pot at a time. A hundred pounds fits easily in the trunk and back seat of a sedan, or in an SUV. And I recently spoke with someone who moves essentially infinite amounts of marijuana from the Emerald Triangle to Louisiana every two weeks. He has a company wholesaling legal agricultural products out of Sacramento. Almonds, walnuts, cherries, and so on. For obvious reasons, he didn't tell me what he ships. Sometimes these containers are full of legal agricultural products, and sometimes they're partially filled with illegal agricultural products.

We've all seen those movies.

A lot of people drive it themselves in their own cars, U-Haul trucks or trailers, or RVs. All of this happens enough to cause police in many states through which the mules must pass to profile vehicles with California tags, certain types of rentals, and RVs, especially those driven by people who aren't senior citizens. I knew one guy who converted his big propane delivery truck to carry grass instead of gas.

The second reason it isn't really accurate is that people have been sending contraband through commercial transportation systems as long as commercial transportation systems have existed.

I just watched a video of a museum curator who is delightfully obsessed with a family of traders from Assyria 4,000 years ago who, fortunately for her and for us, left extensive correspondence via cuneiform tablet. And what, among other things, did they talk about? Smuggling, mainly textiles and tin. There were two primary methods smugglers used to move goods from Anastasia in modern Turkey to Assyria in modern Iraq. The first was to travel the "narrow track"—in other words, avoid the main trade routes with soldiers, tollgates, and customs officials and take hidden paths with bandits, poor maintenance, and wild animals. Using this method, they didn't have to pay tolls and export and import fees. The other method was to follow the conventional route and simply hide the goods to be smuggled, revealing, as always, that not much has changed in the last 4,000 years. One tablet suggests that trading partners can smuggle tin by making sure, just before they enter town, to gather the tin into parcels and put these parcels into their underwear.[2] Revealing again that not much has changed. . .

Now let's move forward 2,500 years—during which, people continued to move goods by narrow tracks and put parcels in their underwear—to 551 CE, when China had had for some 700 years a monopoly on silkworms, and thus silk. This monopoly was remarkably profitable and important for China, so important that the Silk Road trade route was named after it. It was China's primary export. That year, a couple of Nestorian monks who had been preaching the Good News in India made their way to China, where they observed silk worm farms. They saw a great opportunity for smuggling and took off for

---

[2] "A 4,000-year-old tale of trade and contraband: Curator's Corner Season 3 Episode 9," *The British Museum*, March 25, 2018, accessed November 17, 2019, https://www.youtube.com/watch?v=bQIBf7eeXG8.

Constantinople to talk to the Byzantine emperor Justinian I. Justinian was pleased enough to promise them great things if they'd bring him some silkworm eggs. The details of his promises were either kept private or lost through time, but they must have been great indeed, since the penalty for being caught smuggling these eggs was death. Yet the monks returned to China, acquired some eggs, hid them in the hollows of their canes, and smuggled the eggs to Constantinople. Soon the Byzantine Empire established worm farms, and more important to regional commerce, a European silk monopoly that lasted 650 years and an industry that has lasted until today.

One person's smuggling is another person's commercial theft is another person's business opportunity.

Entire regional economies have been based on the movement of contraband using commercial transportation systems. After the English Civil War, and to pay for wars thereafter, the British government imposed a series of customs on imported goods and excises on any number of domestic purchases. It also banned certain exports, for example, grain. People responded through widespread smuggling. How widespread? At one point as much as 80 percent of tea drunk in Britain had been smuggled. Most of the gin had also been smuggled. I didn't say "gin drunk in Britain," since smuggled gin was so commonplace that people used it to clean their windows. The economies of south England and the Scilly and Shetland Isles were almost completely dependent on smuggling. It's not too much to say that at times essentially all money in the Shetland Isles was associated with smuggling.

When customs officials seized goods, frequently entire communities rose to seize them back.

Let's talk about North America.

Using commercial transportation systems to move contraband was essential to the runup to the American Revolution and, indeed, to funding it. In attempts to force American colonists to buy British goods, the Crown passed acts like the Molasses Act, renewed as the Sugar Act, and various Navigation acts, putting high duties on goods imported from other than British territories. These acts were largely ignored by colonists, and any attempts at British enforcement increased colonists' resentment. Those who were caught by the British were often let off by juries of their peers. This led to the British trying prisoners by judges only—British, of course—which further magnified resentment. These were among the primary reasons Americans eventually rebelled. Further, skills learned by smugglers were critical to American war efforts.

All of which is to say that one person's smuggling can be another person's treason can be another person's patriotism.

Let's move forward to some other examples of shipping contraband, in these cases definitely not patriotic, through commercial or institutional means of transportation.

During the Vietnam War a lot of US soldiers used military transports to move heroin bought in Thailand for $4,000/kg to the United States, where it would be cut four times and sold for $100,000/kg. They moved it in hollowed-out furniture, in parcels—you name it. There were rumors, probably untrue, that they moved it in caskets of soldiers killed in Vietnam.

The point is that they used US military transports to move their contraband.

Next story: I have a friend who has a friend who has a friend—so three degrees of separation—who founded a business moving ambulances from Florida, where they were manufactured, up to New England, where he would sell them. There is some money to be made in transporting ambulances, I suppose. But the real money came from packing the spaces inside panels with cocaine, which would be removed on arrival and sold. He only got caught because he made an enemy of his wife, who turned him in.

Looking to verify this story, I searched for the words "ambulance," "cocaine," and "smuggling," and found to my surprise—although in retrospect I should be surprised at my surprise—that he was either a trendsetter or a copycat, because evidently smuggling via ambulances is not uncommon, as I immediately saw news articles spanning the globe, from the UK to Thailand, of people using ambulances to smuggle drugs.

I also saw articles about people using pineapples, submarines, office furniture, hollowed-out crucifixes, and on and on and on in order to smuggle contraband.

I used to know someone who knew someone who did undercover work for the Humane Society, making sure shrimpers in the Gulf of Mexico used turtle-excluder-devices (TEDs) on their shrimp nets. TEDs can be cumbersome and can reduce nets' effectiveness at catching shrimp, and since most people don't care about wild nature, shrimpers often won't use them and will then drown sea turtles as bycatch in their nets. His job was to work on a boat, document whether the shrimper was or wasn't using TEDs, and then facilitate the arrest of the shrimper. The friend of a friend had been assembling evidence on one particular shrimp boat for a while, and it was determined that the shrimper would be busted when he next returned to Galveston.

So far, so good.

But shrimpers and fishermen in the Gulf of Mexico sometimes make unreported stops to pick up cocaine and bring it to the US. Heck, shrimpers and fishermen are known around the world for transporting contraband. I know someone in Crescent City, in far northern California, who worked for a fisherman who had a gambling problem, got in debt to the wrong people, and in order to get out from under the debt had to make a run all the way down the coast to Mexico to pick up some cocaine, put it into weighted containers they could haul on lines behind the boat (to be cut loose if they got hailed by the Coast Guard), and brought back home.

So, on the run where the shrimper was going to be busted for not using his TEDs, he decided to smuggle some cocaine. This was terrible news for the guy working undercover, because the penalty for not using TEDs was a fairly small fine, and the shrimper would only be moderately pissed at him. The penalty for smuggling cocaine would be years in prison for the shrimper, and the lifelong enmity of a cocaine cartel for the guy working undercover. He tried desperately to get the shrimper to call off the smuggling during that run, and tried just as desperately to get officials to call off the bust. Neither worked, and as soon as the boat landed, and after he'd been faux-arrested along with the real arrestees, then quietly released, he got the hell out of Texas, never to return.

Let's bring this back to using the mails for contraband. Have you ever gotten spam advertising Vi.Ag.Ra? Of course you have, unless you have an impregnable spam filter, because 65 percent of all spam is for pharmaceuticals.

Fifteen years ago I responded to one. Well, not for Vi.Ag.Ra, of course. Harrumph, I would never need that. And truth be told, I didn't quite respond to a spam, but close enough. And don't worry, I'm still paying for my sin.

I had an infection. I'd had a similar infection the year before and the doctor had recommended doxycycline. This was before Obamacare, and as a freelance writer I didn't have health insurance. I didn't want to pay money I didn't have for an office visit just to get a prescription. So I went online and ordered doxycycline from an Indian pharmacy. Like the superballs on eBay the pills were cheaper in quantity, so I got a hundred, even though I only needed ten.

I was at the time a little concerned that I was going to get in trouble for ordering contraband through the mail. I pictured someone from customs and immigration coming to my door, cuffs at the ready. Then I got a notice in my mailbox that I had a parcel at the post office. I decided that's where they were going to pop me. I put my affairs in order, arranged for someone to take care of my animals if the worst transpired, then went to the post office. I live in a tiny town, so the postal clerks smiled and welcomed me by name. One said, "We've got something for you."

I watched to see if the other reached under the counter to press some sort of silent alarm.

The first walked into another room, took a suspiciously long time.

I figured he was stalling till the cops got there.

Finally, he came back, carrying a five-by-eight envelope. He gave the envelope a little shake. We both heard the rattling of pills. He flipped me a smile that said he knew I was buying diamond-shaped blue pills.

I wanted to shout out, "I'm not buying Vi.Ag.Ra," but I presumed they'd all figure I was protesting too much.

So my walk on the wild side did not cost me time in the big house. It did, however, cost me in another way. Surprisingly enough, the company did not steal my credit card information. They did, however, sell my information to God knows how many pharmaceutical companies, because in the fifteen years since then I have received almost daily phone calls asking if I am ready to refill my prescription. I got another call today.

The point, insofar as there is one, is that lots of contraband is sent using the postal service, FedEx, and United Parcel Service. Several years ago UPS was fined $40 million because, as the Department of Justice (DOJ) noted, "Despite being on notice that [illegal] internet pharmacies were using its services, UPS did not implement procedures to close the accounts of those pharmacies, permitting them to ship controlled substances and prescription drugs."[3] For a time, until the case was suddenly dropped, the DOJ had been attempting to fine FedEx $1.6 billion for conspiracy to traffic illegal drugs—both prescription and street. In an article entitled "Is FedEx America's No. 1 Drug Dealer?" *The Daily Beast* describes how, "In a move that the DEA and FDA suggest shows both knowledge of the illicit online pharmacy industry and awareness of its potential for boom and bust, FedEx established an 'Online Pharmacy Credit Policy.' This required all online pharmacies to provide FedEx with a security deposit, bank letter of credit, and to be subjected to 'limited credit terms.' In 2004, the DEA estimated that FedEx had 200 registered online pharmacies. By 2010, it had more than 600." The article quotes a former FedEx employee who, "when he approached his manager with his suspicions about Scotto's [a heroin trafficker's] merchandise in the late 80s, he said he was sternly told that keeping the drug dealer's packages safe was part of his job.

---

[3] "Attachment A," *Department of Justice*, accessed December 1, 2019, https://www.justice.gov/sites/default/files/usao-ndca/legacy/2013/03/29/UPS.AttachmentA.pdf page 8.

'Many times, I have heard a FedEx courier or member of FedEx management boast that, "We're the number one shipper of illegal drugs in America."'[4]

Please note that the feds suddenly dropped the case just as it was going to trial.

It's possible no one has ever shipped contraband using FedEx.

Or. . .

I asked a wholesaler what he's learned about using the mails. He said, "At first I used UPS, until I lost a couple of packages in a row at a store. After the first one disappeared, I figured a store employee got wise and stole it, but after the second one I called about the package not appearing on tracking. The employee asked for the tracking number, and when I gave it, responded, 'Oh, that was turned over to law enforcement.' I hung up the phone, threw it away—it was a burner anyhow—and never went back in that store. Then I started using USPS. The biggest problem I've found is that I can no longer mail large packages that go through the San Francisco sorting center."

"Because of seizures?"

"Of a kind. Thefts. Clearly there's someone or some group of people in that particular sorting center that opens random packages out of northern California, and if it's Grandma Jo sending a sweater to Granddaughter Lisa just re-seals it, no harm done, but if it's five pounds of pot, he's just made himself from 5 to 10K.

"And not only do these thefts cost me money, they're also a pain in the ass, because this means for big shipments I have to drive a hundred miles each way from Arcata, California, to Brookings, Oregon, to mail the damn thing. Packages out of Brookings are sorted in Portland, which for now at least has fewer thieves in their sorting center."

I talked to another wholesaler, asked him if any of the people he mailed to had ever been arrested.

[4] Abby Haglage, "Is FedEx America's No. 1 Drug Dealer?" *Daily Beast*, July 29, 2014, updated April 14, 2017, accessed December 1, 2019, https://www.thedaily-beast.com/is-fedex-americas-no-1-drug-dealer.

He said, "Well, yes and no. Mailing is pretty safe. I've known three who've been arrested, but nobody's gotten in trouble solely over pot."

I had no idea what he was talking about.

He said, "The first one got arrested over pot, but not over mailing. And him getting arrested saved his life."

"Somebody was going to kill him or something?"

"Nothing so dramatic. He and I had a great working relationship, made a lot of money for both of us. He had good outlets and would take everything and anything I could send him, from top of the line to stuff that was barely better than trim. The market was insatiable. He paid off his student debt and bought himself a house.

"At one point one of his buyers ripped him off. If it had happened to me, I would have just written it off. Hell, I've done exactly that. But he thought he needed to beat the guy up to show everyone that nobody gets by with stealing from him. He knew the guy was going to be at a certain bar, so he parked a few blocks away, went in, and punched the guy out. He got arrested for the bar fight, which wasn't a big deal, but he'd left his car in a school zone, so it got impounded the next day. Worse, he'd left several pounds of pot in his trunk, so when the cops found that they gave him a big hassle."

"How did this save his life?"

"He got a concussion in the fight, so from the jail they escorted him to the hospital for a CT scan. The scan revealed a brain tumor. I always wondered if the brain tumor played a part in the cops dropping all charges, since I'm presuming the state would have had to pay for the surgery if he was in custody. In any case he retired after that.

"The next was another guy I made a lot of money with. We were doing great, probably moving a few pounds a week—which converted to $300–400/week profit for me, and I don't know how much for him—when he got greedy."

"Did he steal from you?"

"No, not at all. But he knew somebody who knew somebody who knew somebody who had a connection who could get him MDMA or some other shit from China, and he ordered something like 100,000 pills. The pills got seized at customs and he got sentenced to seven years in the federal pen. It's too bad, since we could still be grinding away and both of us paying our rent. Although come to think of it, he doesn't have to pay rent right now."

"And the third?"

"He was moving about ten pounds a week, so $1,000 a week profit for me. We'd been doing this for a few years. I was able to put all that money away. It was a good scene. It started to fall apart when my connection, let's call him Dave, knew that another dealer in his town was beating the shit out of his girlfriend. So Dave went to the cops about the violence. He never mentioned the other guy was a dealer, just that he was violent. The cops went to talk to the abuser, but of course didn't do anything. The perp, however, knew who had gone to the cops and retaliated by telling the cops Dave was a dealer who received pot through the mail. The next shipment was intercepted at the post office, and law enforcement did what's called a controlled delivery: an officer pretended to be a postal employee and took the package to Dave's house. Dave accepted the package. The cops arrested Dave and asked if they could search his house. He said no. They took him away, but he denied any knowledge of why anyone would send him marijuana."

"Ah, the Gilligan defense."

He stared at me.

"In the late nineties, Bob Denver, who played Gilligan on Gilligan's Island . . ."

"*Little Buddy!*"

". . . was arrested for receiving a package of marijuana in the mail. He claimed Dawn Wells sent it to him . . ."

"*Mary Ann sent Gilligan some pot?* Well, that explains a lot about that show."

". . . but then refused to name her in court, saying instead that for reasons unknown to him some 'crazy fan' had sent him the marijuana."

"Yeah, that's always the best defense. The cops can hassle you, but if they only catch you once, and it's not something outrageous like 100,000 pills, you can just deny knowledge of it. Dave went to an attorney, who told him to do exactly that. The attorney said, 'The moment you walk out of here, clean your house. Get rid of all drugs, all money, you name it. And whatever you do, don't allow anyone to send you any more pot for a couple of months. If you keep your house clean for that long, the cops will drop it. They honestly don't give a shit about marijuana.'

"So he and I paused our business. That should have been fine. But what I didn't know is that in addition to selling pot, he was using and selling heroin. And the guy really was an addict. He couldn't keep that shit out of his house even for two months. The cops came back with a search warrant a few weeks later, found his heroin stash and his needles and everything else.

"He had no money for bail or even to pay that attorney to represent him for more than that one visit. While I'd been putting money away for my retirement—I don't even smoke pot, for God's sake—he was shooting up every bit of profit. They charged him with intent to distribute both marijuana and heroin. He was facing a long time.

"There's something interesting about the marijuana charge. For whatever reason, that week I'd only sent him two pounds of pot. But pot is pretty lightweight, so to disguise it and keep both cops and thieves from profiling the packages and opening them, each for their own reasons, I include baseball-sized rocks in the packages. But because the package weighed ten pounds, the cops were charging him with possession of ten pounds of pot. Clearly bullshit."

"Cop shenanigans with evidence reminds me of a story told me by someone I know. Decades ago, he distributed cocaine in Florida. He also used a lot. He's clean now and also would never sell it anymore. He's turned over such a new leaf that he won't even speed anymore. I met him because he picked me up at the airport to deliver me to a talk I was doing. My flight was delayed, and unless we hurried, I was going to be late for my own event. But the needle refused to cross the magical 55 mph mark.

"In those earlier days his cocaine use was making him paranoid, and he was more or less always certain cops were about to bust in his door and arrest him. But one of those hallucinations was true, and they did bust in his door, caught him trying to flush everything he had down the toilet. Enough remained unflushed to put him away for decades.

But when the charges were drawn up and presented, the amount of cocaine was off by a factor of ten in his favor. It made no difference to him and his attorney whether this was some sort of clerical error or whether some corrupt cop had stolen 90 percent of his cocaine. They both leapt to their feet and couldn't plead guilty fast enough.

"Maybe his refusal to speed is the result of one of those bargains we so often make with God or Fate *in extremis* but that never seem to come to fruition: 'If you make it so most of this goes away, I will never again break a law for the rest of my life. And I even promise to floss my teeth.'"

The wholesaler responded, "In my guy's case he sat in jail for months while the DA, his public defender, and the judge tried to figure out a plea deal. The DA was a big animal-rights activist, so he floated the idea that if Dave gave 15K to an animal shelter, they'd all call it good. As with the guy you knew in Florida, Dave couldn't sign off on that one fast enough—I could have lent him the money if he would have stayed off the smack—but the judge nixed it. I don't remember what the final settlement was, but he stayed in for a couple of years. And remember, he wouldn't have spent even one night in jail if it weren't for the heroin."

"This all sounds like, frankly, a pretty dangerous way to make a living."

"It does, from just these stories, but you have to understand I've been doing this for thirty years, with scores of business partnerships lasting a few months to a couple of decades, and in all that time only three of them have been arrested. And again, none of them got in trouble for pot. Mostly the business part of this is just tedious. Lots of sourcing pot, getting friends to test it for me, then hour after hour vacuum sealing, packing it in mylar, and visiting every post office within a hundred miles.

"Something else people need to understand is that the margin on marijuana isn't that great. There's a cliché that drugs have the biggest markup of any product. That may be true for hard drugs, but it's just not true for marijuana. At every step of the process, margins are low to middling. Maybe back when marijuana was $3,000 or more a pound, but when indoor growers are getting from $1,500 to $2,000/lb., they're only making a few hundred a pound profit. And my markup is generally about $100/lb., which is crap. It sounds like it's a lot, because you can't make $100/lb. on tomatoes, but then again, the farm price of tomatoes is something like fifty cents a pound with a retail markup of about 100 to 200 percent, depending on where you are. So if you go by money invested and not pounds, suddenly marijuana doesn't seem so great an investment. The reason I've been able to make a lot of money at it is that the demand is essentially infinite. And also, I've worked really hard.

"The great thing about marijuana, and the reason illegal grows in many ways represented the American Dream, is that the barriers to entry were so small. Almost anyone could do it. I've known outdoor growers who started with a few plants in a guerilla grow, where they didn't even own the land, and then sold the pot from those plants, and slowly built up—and indoor growers who started with a grow in their closet, with startup expenses of a few hundred dollars, and increased over time. And I've known wholesalers who started with enough money to buy one pound of pot, sold it, and used that money to buy another pound, until they'd accumulated enough to buy two pounds, then three, then four. There aren't really that many businesses you can start with such a small initial investment. And because of the illegality you don't have to deal with multiple layers of bureaucracy.

"I've talked to illegal growers and distributors who since legalization wanted to enter the aboveground market. They've consistently been told that if you don't have a couple hundred thousand dollars in ready cash, don't bother.

"Times have changed.

"But there's another problem here that we all face, which is that the illegality brings a lot more risk. Not just of arrest, but also of theft, and of having no safety net, no insurance if things go wrong. There have been years where I have a few good buyers and no thefts, and I make really good money. But then someone at the postal sorting facility steals a ten-pound package, and I'm out the $15,000 I paid to the grower. And then the week after, a new buyer rips me off for another ten pounds, and I'm out another $15,000. And the week after that, I buy ten pounds from a grower who doesn't deliver, and I'm out another $15,000. There have been stretches of two or three years where I've done nothing but lose money. A lot of money. Being in this business has taught me, if nothing else, to be a good and conservative money manager."

I said, "I know an outdoor grower right on the border with Oregon—"

"Uh-oh."

"Why do you say that?"

"Because a lot of outdoor growers in or near Oregon are in bad shape."

Oregon recently legalized industrial hemp. Hemp is cannabis with extremely low THC. It's grown for multiple reasons, including extracting CBD, or cannabidiol, the second-most abundant cannabinoid in pot, which happens to be non-intoxicating and can help with inflammation, anxiety, pain, and seizures. As a consequence of legalization, massive fields of industrial hemp have been planted all over Oregon.

If you recall, marijuana is sexually dimorphic. The buds people smoke come only from unfertilized female plants. Fertilized plants put their energy into seeds—as they should—rather than into THC. And I've heard people say, though never experienced it myself, that smoking seeds gives you a headache. Just a few seeds can cause buyers to reject an entire pound of pot. And cannabis is wind-pollinated, with the males able to fertilize females more than seven miles away. When the wind is right, male plants in Morocco can pollinate female plants thirty miles away, in Spain.

I said, "The guy grew a hundred pounds, and it all got pollinated by a hemp field somewhere on the other side of the border. He had no idea the other field was there."

"Jesus wept," the distributor said.

"So did this grower," I responded. If we figure $800/lb. for outdoor, this was an $80,000 loss after he'd put in the time and expense to grow his crop.

*

Theft isn't an issue only for those participating in illegal activities. A few weeks ago I was the third wheel in a conversation between a builder friend and a manager at *The Home Depot*. The manager said that because of the threat of lawsuits by thieves who might claim to have been mishandled while being held till the arrival of police, store policy is to let shoplifters walk out of the store with whatever they want.

My friend asked, "You mean a tweaker can roll out with a generator?"

"Happens all the time. I've seen tweakers roll a generator directly from the display to the returns desk, say they lost their receipt, and try to get cash for it. When we tell them no, they just roll it on out the front door."

I asked, "Why did I just pay for these screws?"

They both ignored me, which was probably for the best.

My friend asked, "Do you at least call the cops?"

"Yes, but by the time they get here the thief is long gone."

"Can you follow them out to the parking lot?"

"Sure, but all we can do is get a license number. And often the tweakers didn't drive a car. They just roll the shit on down the street." He paused a moment and then said, "There are stores in some towns where they lose a couple million dollars a year, and just write it off as a cost of doing business."

Thieves abound.

A few days ago, I got an email from FedEx saying a package I'd ordered had arrived. I looked on the porch: nothing. A while later I walked out to the gate. Nothing. I waited a couple of days, called FedEx, pressed lots of buttons, cursed several times, and finally—and more or less randomly—somehow got to talk to a human. I explained the situation. The representative said the package had been left off at my gate.

And then, evidently, stolen.

Thefts of packages from porches are so common—about 11 million people in the US report this every year—they've spawned a genre of YouTube videos about people putting out decoy packages containing glitter and fart bombs as well as cameras to record and remotely upload videos of the thieves freaking out when they open the stolen packages.

For two years in my 1980s I lived in tiny Carlin, Nevada. Down the street lived a clan of thieves run by a matriarch who was literally, but not figuratively, toothless—meth's way of saying hello. The only good thing is that they didn't steal from their immediate neighbors. Once, a U-Haul someone was using to move cross-country broke down on I-70 just outside of town. Because cell phones wouldn't become commonplace for another fifteen years, the people making the move had to hitchhike the twenty-three miles east to Elko to get a tow truck. It took the clan less than the couple of hours it took for the victims to return in a tow truck for them empty the U-Haul.

Thieves abound.

I've only bought pot twice in my life, and both times I did it legally. My mom was dying of an inoperable and aggressive pancreatic/biliary duct cancer that was far beyond any hope of chemo. We did a Hail Mary and called a doctor in Oregon who specializes in marijuana extracts for cancer. He prescribed some THC and CBD tinctures and suppositories. I paid for them—a few thousand dollars—and because he couldn't ship them across state lines, a friend who was going to be in Oregon picked them up for me.

My first experience buying marijuana wasn't much different than buying some other high-ticket item online.

My mom religiously took the CBD oil, but she didn't like the THC. It made her hallucinate. She would see demons rise up from the edge of the bed and zoom across the ceiling. When she said she would rather die than spend the rest of her time hallucinating about demons, I understood.

We thought maybe the THC oil was too strong, no matter how little I gave her, so I went into a local dispensary and bought a THC-infused chocolate bar.

My second experience wasn't much different than buying a candy bar at a convenience store.

Even tiny slivers of the chocolate still made her hallucinate.

It would be easy to say the marijuana didn't work for my mom. She still suffered from the cancer, and she still died. But to me the tincture was worth every penny, because in the weeks before my mom died, and up until a couple of days before she entered terminal delirium, she would ask me, almost every evening as I administered the CBD oil drops beneath her tongue, "When do you think this is going to start kicking in?"

And even though I knew different, I would say, "Soon. Soon."

The CBD gave her hope in this clearly hopeless situation. I could not put a price on that.

Long after my mom died, I spoke with someone who used to grow, back when it was illegal, but who has been forced out of business by legality. She said, "I've specialized in CBD for a long time, since before it was easy to acquire CBD genetics, and I have so many wonderful stories about people benefiting from CBD. A high school kid being able to go back to school because her seizures were finally stopped completely because of my CBD. A ten-year-old boy was able to play with his eight-year-old old sister for the first time. A single mom who struggled with debilitating Crohn's for forty years experienced her first day of relief ever with CBD. She asked to meet me, so I drove four hours. I will never forget standing in her driveway hugging her and crying with her. The local psychiatric facility approved CBD to be included in medication protocols. A woman contacted me after my business was destroyed and told me my CBD got her out of a wheelchair from an autoimmune disease, but since legality, the stuff she buys in stores doesn't work. I've heard so many stories like that. Honestly, now that industry got a hold of CBD, the mass-produced products are not nearly as good. I would say 95 percent of them are absolute crap. Low quality genetics, farmed with low quality standards, extracted with low quality or harmful solvents, then mixed with low quality oils that have been subject to the same processes, packaged in fancy containers and marketed with expensive advertising in order to minimize cost and maximize profit."

I don't know how end-user illegal marijuana sales work. I was such a nerd all through high school and college that I rarely witnessed any sort of marijuana action.

Actually, that's not fair to nerds. Being a nerd myself, I was privy to the fact that a lot of nerds use a lot of drugs. They just generally have wordier and more intellectual (although sometimes pithy) rationalizations for their drug use than do most people, as they generally have wordier and more intellectual (although sometimes pithy) rationalizations for many of the things they do.

It is, however, fair to me. I have only three memories of anything having to do with end-user illegal marijuana sales up to the age of, well, I was going to say up to the end of my thirties, but the truth is it's to this day.

The first was when I was sixteen, walking with a friend in Denver on a brisk fall afternoon.

A man walking in the other direction asked us quietly, "Wanna get high?"

I smiled, as only a nerd can smile—and that's not a compliment—then said, "I'm already high, man. Ask me how high."

The guy's face was resigned. He said, flatly, "How high?"

"Fifty-two hundred and eighty feet, man. Mile High Denver."

The man shook his head in disgust as my friend and I high-fived.

Yes, as a teenager I was a nerd. Oh, who'm I kidding? I'm still a nerd. I'm a writer, so the only way I could be a worse nerd is if I had a degree in something nerdy like physics. Oops.

I also saw various drug transactions at rock concerts. I remember wondering at the audacity of a man standing within ten feet of a cop outside the Red Rocks Amphitheater near Morrison, Colorado, before a Blue Öyster Cult show, saying softly to anyone who walked by, "Hash? Hash?" I also remember wondering if the guy had already sampled too much of his own product, to think anyone was going to buy from him that close to a police officer.

I also remember going home from the concert astounded at the wonderful light show the band put on. Not being nerds or anything, my friends and I did not try to put on our own version of "Laser Rock" by tightly taping reflective mylar over the front of a woofer, cranking up the volume, and bouncing a laser beam off the vibrating surface. In public. Having advertised the idea without first testing it. Had we done this, and we most certainly did not, the audience of 1970s teen-agers—even though they were as yet unjaded by computers, and for whom Pong, Asteroids, and Advent were the height of technological entertainment—would nonetheless not have been so unimpressed as to leave after only a few minutes. And if they had, I would of course not harbor a bitterness about it to this day.

My third experience of attempted illegal marijuana retail exchange happened in my thirties, when I lived in Spokane, Washington. I was waiting at the shop for my car to be fixed, when another customer came in to the waiting room, sat next to me, said, "I'm from out of town," then asked earnestly, "How green is my valley?"

"I'm sorry?" I responded.

He repeated his question.

My first thought was that he was lost. There's a suburb of Spokane locally called The Valley. I said, "When your car's fixed, get on the interstate, go east a ways, and you should see lots of exit signs."

He shook his head, asked again, this time slowly emphasizing each word as though I were dim, "How green is my valley?"

This time I thought he was referring to the 1940s John Ford film of nearly the same name. I couldn't for the life of me figure out why he'd be asking me about that movie. It's not a bad movie but has nothing to do with automobile repair. Maybe he's a Maureen O'Hara fan? Maybe he's still mad it beat out *Citizen Kane* for best movie that year? I shook my head slightly.

He asked it again, even more earnestly than before.

This time I thought, is he coming on to me? He's from out of town and wants a one-night stand? After all, the title of the book on which the movie was based comes from the main character reflecting imme-diately after his first sexual experience, "How green was my Valley that day, too, green and bright in the sun." Was this a come-on with built-in literary gatekeeping, to prevent those who aren't well-read from getting his meaning? Or was "valley" some reference to my behind? But what does "green" mean in that context? Does he want someone inexperienced? But he said "my valley." Maybe he's saying *his* behind is green, *he* is inexperienced. Maybe that's why his come-on is simultaneously vague and oddly specific. That had to be it. It's the only thing that made sense. I said to him, "I'm not gay, but you're really sweet to offer. I'm flattered."

He stared at me hard, this time using his eyes rather than his enunciation to show he considered me dim. Then he looked stealthily around the room and asked it one more time, before making the universal hand-gesture for toking. Thumb and forefinger pressed tightly together, then brought to his mouth, cheeks pulling in as he sucked air through pursed lips.

"Oh, I get it!" I said. "Sorry, I don't smoke."

I later asked a stoner friend if I was, as always, hopelessly naïve, and this was part of the marijuana subculture argot to which I'd never been initiated.

He said, "Nah. The guy was just nuts."

That made me feel a little better.

I used to teach creative writing in a prison. Many of my students were, in one way or another, in because of drugs—from minimum security students in for simple possession or burglary to support a drug habit, to supermax students in for killing people in drug deals gone bad or even for being hit men who had killed for $500 a pop to support their habits.

A primary reason I became a writer, and *the* primary reason I became a physicist, is because I love learning how things work. I often think I'm addicted to the steep part of the learning curve. And one reason I do so many interviews is that I love learning from people who know more than I do. Put these together, and I probably learned more from my students than they learned from me.

For example, many told me that if you dropped them in any major city in the United States, they'd be able to find drugs in less than half an hour.

In many cities, it would take me that long to find a parking space.

Many told me the competition is fierce among drug dealers, often but not always leading to tremendous customer service. They said if they ordered pizza and cocaine at the same time, the cocaine would probably arrive first.

They also told me—and I know you'll be shocked by this—that while *The Shawshank Redemption* may have been a good movie, it was terribly unrealistic. One inaccuracy was that Red added a 20 percent surcharge to have items smuggled into prison. My students told me the going rate for contraband is not 20 percent higher than street value, but ten times street value. If a gram of marijuana goes for $10 outside, it would be $100 inside.

I asked how most drugs are smuggled into prison. It's easy in minimum security, they said, since the fence is chain link and things can be easily thrown over. Where I taught, the handball wall was near a fence, and when I'd park then walk to the classroom I'd routinely pick up the half-dozen balls that had accidentally cleared the fence and toss them back over, or give them to my supervisor to hand back out. Evidently, some people sneak into the parking lot and toss over bags of drugs. Presumably, the price is lower in minimum security than in supermax because of the ease of smuggling.

In higher levels some types of drugs like LSD can be sent hidden in the mail, for example behind a design on a card. Prison employees open every piece of mail and handle every page to make sure nothing is stuck to it. Visitors also bring in some drugs. One way is through putting drugs in a condom and putting it in your rectum, called "packing the trunk," then once in the visiting area, entering the restroom, removing the condom, putting the condom in your pocket, and at some point removing it and passing it to the prisoner, who repeats the process in reverse. See, people are still smuggling things inside their underwear, although admittedly this takes it a step further. Because of this, at many prisons—on the way from the visiting room back to the yard—the prisoner will have to drop trousers, squat, spread cheeks, and cough.

But by far the main channel for smuggling drugs into prison, they told me, is guards. The 1,000 percent markup evidently overrides other considerations, including loss of job and potential loss of freedom, even though pay for guards starts upwards of 50K, not bad for a job requiring only a high school education.

It wouldn't be that difficult for a guard to smuggle. The first couple of times I went in they looked carefully through my bag, but after that the search was pretty *pro forma*, and I didn't even go in during shift change. There wouldn't be enough time to ask all the guards to turn out their pockets. And a person could keep a lot of contraband in those pockets.

Several students told me how a typical interaction might work. After a series of preliminary conversations where each side feels out the other, a prisoner might ask, "How are the Christmas trees this year?"

"There are a lot of them if you know where to look."

"My family deserves a nice, top-quality Christmas tree. How much do those run these days?"

The guard would name a price.

"Where would my family send the money?"

The guard would name a PO box.

When the cash arrived, the guard would bring in the contraband.

Prisoners suggested the guard might put a couple of joints in a nearly empty snack bag of potato chips, then walk near the inmate, pull out the last couple of chips, look in the bag, throw it on the ground like it's trash, and walk away. The inmate would pick up the bag, mime throwing it in the trash, and the transfer would be complete.

I'm sure in some prisons, guards could just hand the contraband to the prisoners when they're out of sight of a camera, but the prison I taught at was a panopticon design, so it presumably would have been a bit more difficult to be out of view of surveillance cameras or other guards.

But 1,000-percent markup can make people awfully creative.

A couple of prisoners asked me to bring them in some marijuana. Not even remotely tempted, I turned them down flat.

I had of course never shared with them that I grow. Standard prison policy strongly discourages telling prisoners anything about your life. Once, a student asked what I was doing for Thanksgiving, and I responded that I was spending it with my mom. My supervisor took me aside afterwards and said even that amount of sharing was inadvisable, since you never know how someone might try to use information against you. That seemed a bit strict, but I could easily see why telling criminals—many of whom were involved in gangs both in and out of prison—that I grew small amounts of marijuana would be a terrible idea.

They nonetheless asked, as I presumed they asked whomever seemed even slightly sympathetic or gullible. Or maybe they mistook my act of listening to their stories about their lives as a willingness to do more than listen.

At first, I didn't consider their request long enough to even bother asking myself why I found the idea preposterous. It just seemed like a Terrible Idea. I have in my life made manifest many Terrible Ideas—from jumping off a roof as a kid since it seemed to work fine for those who did it in movies; to, in my teens and early twenties, not bothering to scrape the ice off the windshield but driving hunched over looking through the bottom inch as the defroster slowly did its thing; to any number of unwise and unprofitable business ventures since then; to God knows what idiocy I'm doing now. If I could name it as a Terrible Idea in real time, I probably wouldn't do it, right? But smuggling drugs into a super-maximum- security prison to hand them to potential gang members seemed to me to be the Babe Ruth of Terrible Ideas, the Elvis Presley of Terrible Ideas, the Nobel Prize Winner in the category of Terrible Ideas.

Obviously, there are a great number of people who don't think this is a Terrible Idea, since they routinely smuggle everything from LSD to marijuana, to cell phones, to chargers into even supermax prisons. So I've often in the time since wondered why I wasn't tempted when so many other people are.

The first reason is that it's illegal. I know that sounds odd in the middle of a book about the culture of illegal marijuana, but smuggling something into a super-maximum-security prison seems a lot more dangerous than growing small amounts of pot in a region world-famous for exactly that.

One of the things Tim and Mario said that helped convince me it was safe to grow in the first place is that not only were most small growers protected by Prop 215—unless you're mixing guns and growing or other drugs and growing—but you're also probably going to get one "get-out-of-jail-free" card. Cops have too many other things to do to waste much time on small growers.

I've seen confirmation of this many times. Years ago I got a frantic email from someone whom I had never before heard from, but who had read my work, saying she and her boyfriend had been arrested here in Crescent City with pot in their car and were facing many years in prison. She asked if I could help. I wrote her back to say I wasn't sure what I could do, since I didn't know any attorneys or have any other special resources I could offer. She wrote me back a couple of days later to say it was all fine, that all charges had been dropped, and they'd merely had their pot confiscated.

Also many years ago, right after I'd started growing, some young people were evidently wandering through the forest and came upon my house. I wasn't there. At the time I didn't even lock my door; living in the forest, the only reason I even closed my door was to keep bears out. When I got home the door was open. Nothing was gone so I figured I'd forgotten to shut it, or that bears had slid the glass door open. I've seen them do this. But I realized it had been humans when a couple of days later I came home to find the door open again, and stuff missing. I didn't much mind what they stole, since I was at that point still the worst grower in the world, and what they stole was a big box of moldy pot that I'd been trying to figure out what to do with. If we leave aside the violation, they really just solved a disposal problem for me.

But they came back, and came back again, and again, a couple of times a week. I started locking my doors, of course, and I bought some home surveillance cameras. I discovered that the thieves would be waiting in the forest, watching for me to leave, and would come in a few minutes later. Note to anyone reading this: sliding glass door locks are useless against any experienced thief. By jerking on the door in just the right way, the thieves easily popped the locks. They carried bats and wore ski masks, which they removed as soon as they got in the house. The cameras caught close-ups of their faces.

At the time I had an elderly rescue border collie cross named Shade. He loved me and my mom fiercely for having rescued him and didn't much like anyone else. He normally walked with me when I left my house, but one day his arthritis was especially bothering him, and I was only going to be gone a short while, so I left him. That day the cameras caught them beating Shade with their bats.[5]

That was when I started fantasizing about bear traps, small caliber handguns, and whether it would be best to dump their bodies in the forest to feed bears, in the ocean to feed fish, or in a mineshaft to feed microorganisms.

Instead, I did one of the smartest things I've ever done. I took the video to a friend who worked for someone who'd lived his whole life in Crescent City. It's a small enough community that he recognized one of the people in the video. Then we looked on Facebook, and there he was. Let's click on his friends. Hey, I recognize this guy, and that guy too! And when he's not stealing from people this one works at Wendy's, and that one posts pictures of himself captioned, "Mustache rides, ladies?"

Because they'd stolen pot, I wasn't comfortable going to the sheriff's office. I briefly considered asking tough friends to go to Wendy's and publicly tell that particular thief we knew what he'd done and where he lived. Instead, and somehow the smart decisions continued, I hired a private investigator to represent me to the sheriff's office.

I cannot recommend this highly enough for people who have to go to the police. Just as we need an advocate when the police are coming

---

[5] Shade survived and shared a few more years with me before he crossed the rainbow bridge. When it eventually is my turn, I'll see you on the other side, my friend.

after us, we need an advocate when we want the police to protect us. The investigator told me which detectives in the sheriff's office were lazy and which took their jobs more seriously. He called the best detective for me. He kept pushing the sheriff's department to act until they arrested a couple of the perps.

I bring up this story for a couple of reasons. The first is that a few days after the investigator called the detective, the detective called me. I told him more about what had happened, and he said, "Can I come see the crime scene?"

I said, "Of course. When works?"

"How about right now?"

I knew what he was doing: checking to see if my grow was legal. I brassed it out, "Sounds great. You have my address. Do you need directions?" Of course, I was wondering how many plants I could haul into the forest and hide in the fifteen minutes it would take him to get to my house.

He hesitated a moment, then said, "I think I've got enough from the videos. I don't need to come out."

Suspicion confirmed.

The case eventually ended up at the DA's office, where it sat. And sat. And sat. I finally called to ask what was happening, spoke with an assistant district attorney. She told me they couldn't file any charges because while the alleged thieves said that yes, they had broken into my house, they said they did so only to "hang out."

I said, "If they broke into your house to 'hang out,' would you be so blasé?"

She acknowledged she would not.

"And if they stole from you and beat your dog with sticks?"

"What?"

"Did you not even look at the surveillance video?"

"What surveillance video?"

Eventually the thieves received misdemeanor charges. They were supposed to pay me restitution. One paid about one-fourth of what he was supposed to, the others nothing at all.

While all of this made me feel insecure about police protecting me, it made me feel secure about them not coming after me. Or more or less anyone.

A third confirmation that the legal risk from marijuana is fairly low, unless you're unlucky, came from a conversation I recently overheard at a post office. The customer at the counter next to me was one of those people who, because of low self-esteem or having been abused, feels the need to overdescribe her reasons for doing anything slightly out of the norm. When the clerk couldn't read the addressee's first name, she said, "It's Mayfly. That's not her real name. It's just what everybody calls her."

The clerk smiled and said, "It will get to her."

She said, "Everybody calls her that."

"It's all good."

She continued, "I just didn't want you to think I was using a fake name for her and I'm really sending marijuana through the mail."

All conversation in the post office stopped. Everyone stared at the woman. She started to turn red. Clearly to make her feel better, the clerk said, "People mail marijuana out of this post office every day. We don't have any idea how much is sent, and honestly we don't care."

The point is that while I wasn't much worried about growing small amounts of pot, I strongly suspected the legal system would take a dimmer view of trying to smuggle illegal drugs into one of the most secure prisons in the world.

But evidently, I was wrong. I just looked up the penalty for smuggling drugs into prison, and it isn't that severe: generally two to four years. There are people who have done much longer for possession of marijuana. And smuggling is profitable enough that, far from being deterred by the possibility of confinement, people are swallowing condoms full of drugs then intentionally getting arrested so when they shit out the drugs they can sell them inside. Or they are sticking them up their rectums. Recently thirty-five members of the Mexican Mafia were arrested in San Bernardino in a scheme to do just this. One of them had 43 grams of meth, 50 grams of heroin, 5 syringes, and 20 packets of the opiate Suboxone packed in his trunk.[6] Evidently this is common enough that the Los Angeles County Jail now uses electronic wands to detect contraband inside inmates' bodies.

To me at least, this still seems like a Terrible Idea. One of the training films I watched before I started teaching had to do with not putting yourself in a position to be blackmailed by inmates. If you bring them contraband and they can maintain any sort of proof of this, they have you in a position where they can coerce you into bringing more, not only by threatening to expose your relationship but also by threatening physical violence. In fact, multiple defense attorney websites list "you feared for your life if you did not cooperate" as one of the potential defenses used against prosecution for smuggling contraband into prison. And remember the friend of a friend of a friend rule: your friend in prison may or may not be reliable, but what about his friends, and their friends, and then all of their enemies? Many of my students told me that prison is a lot like elementary or junior high, in that a lot of terribly maladjusted people have a lot of time on their hands and are looking for not-very-mature ways to fill that time. Consequently, there's a lot of gossiping, backbiting, scheming, and trying to harm other people for no good reason other than because you can. In other words, it's a lot like what happens among faculty at any major university, among radical political activists, or for that matter on Facebook. Only it's remotely possible those in prison might have, if you can believe it, even fewer scruples.

I've been thinking lately about the morality or immorality of smuggling contraband into prison; smuggling in general; and more broadly, drug (especially marijuana) production or distribution.

I'll say again—for those in the back who've been checking phones, smoking pot, or both—that I think smuggling drugs into prison is a

---

[6] Cindy Von Quendnow and Chris Wolfe, "35 'Foot Soldiers' for Mexican Mafia Charged in Scheme to Smuggle Drugs Hidden in Their Bodies Into San Bernardino Co. Jails," *KTLA5*, April 25, 2019, accessed December 14, 2019, https://ktla.com/2019/04/25/24-suspected-gang-members-and-associates-suspected-of-smuggling-drugs-into-san-bernardino-county-jails/.

Terrible Idea. Me asking about the morality is just me asking about the morality.[7]

There are those who argue that immorality is unimportant, that what's important is illegality, and because smuggling—into prison, across national borders, or anywhere else—is illegal, it should never be done.

But consider this, from an article entitled, "British POW kept in touch with Japanese camp guard for 64 years": "He [the guard Hayato Hirano] showed us kindness and would smuggle in extra food for us. On a cold day, he came in with pasties and other small foodstuffs which his wife had made." The prisoners so appreciated this guard that after Japan's surrender, they traveled to his home to give him and his family food parcels and stayed in contact for the rest of their lives.[8]

Or we can talk about the statement by US seaman Robert O'Brien, who was taken prisoner when Guam was captured by Japan in 1941. He said Japanese soldiers forced American soldiers to run a gauntlet where they were hit by gun butts or bayonets. Then the soldiers were stripped naked and made to lie in the sun. "Before the day was over, they herded us into a building and permitted us to get back some clothes and then the next day we were all locked up in the Cathedral and served two skimpy meals a day. A few brave Guamanians managed to smuggle in a little food and medicine."[9]

Were these Guamanians committing an immoral act? Should they not have done it? From the perspective of the Japanese military, what they did was illegal and probably immoral. From the perspective of the Guamanians and the prisoners, it was illegal yet moral.

POWs at Cabanatuan in the Philippines were forced to work outside the camp to help the Japanese war effort. They'd have starved had

---

[7] I shared this section with a grower who responded, "The moral question I ask about growing pot is, 'Do I or do I not feed my child?'"

[8] William Hollingworth, "British POW kept in touch with Japanese camp guard for 64 years," *Japan Times*, May 25, 2010, accessed December 21, 2019, https://www.japantimes.co.jp/news/2010/05/25/national/history/british-pow-kept-in-touch-with-japanese-camp-guard-for-64-years/#.Xf3lnEdKg2x.

[9] Robert O'Brien, quoted in "WWII: Prisoners Sent to Japan," *Guampedia*, accessed December 21, 2019, https://www.guampedia.com/wwii-prisoners-of-war-sent-to-japan/.

they not received food smuggled into the prison. Guess where smugglers often hid the food? Yes, in their underwear.

I'm not saying smuggling meth into a prison is morally the same as smuggling food into a POW camp. I'm just saying that smuggling itself, even into a prison, is not in every case immoral.

And the morality of smuggling isn't even necessarily defined by what's being smuggled: Irena Sedler was a Polish nurse in World War II who used her job as a social worker checking for typhus in the Warsaw Ghetto to smuggle in food and medicine and to smuggle out children to places with people who would hide them. She was captured, but as she was being detained, she was able to slip the list of children and their homes to a friend who hid the list in her loose clothing. Irena was tortured but refused to give up the names. Later, guards transporting her to be executed were bribed to release her. Her boss, who sounds like the best boss in the world, tried to talk the Germans into reinstating her with back pay. Sedler thought it better to remain in hiding.

In this case, smuggling children was moral.

On the other hand, 1.2 million children are trafficked each year for sexual and other forms of exploitation, with 17,000 of these child slaves smuggled into the United States.

Smuggling children (or women, or men) to exploit them is immoral, and those who do it should have nine grams of lead parked behind the ear.

So it's not even necessarily what one is smuggling that defines its morality.

Then there are those who argue that the *only* problem with smuggling is its illegality. Since smuggling is the prohibited movement of goods or people, to eliminate smuggling you just need to eliminate prohibitions against the movement of goods or people. This removal by definition eliminates all smuggling.

But that's like saying, since murder is defined as unlawful killing, removing laws against murder would reduce the murder rate to zero. Literally true, but not necessarily best for either society or individuals.

And I'm not making up an absurd argument. There are those who argue that since strictures against homosexuality are wrong, all prohibitions against all forms of sex are wrong, including prohibitions against pedophilia, parent/child incest, and bestiality. This is routinely taught by academics at some of the most prestigious universities in the world, who argue that the harm comes not from these sex acts themselves but from social stigma against pedophilia, parent/child incest, and bestiality. No, I'm not kidding.

As concerns drugs, there are those who likewise argue that the harms don't come from the drugs themselves, but from proscriptions against them. Again, I'm not making this up: at a 2016 Libertarian Party presidential debate, some people booed when candidate Austin Petersen stated, "You should not be able to sell heroin to a five-year-old."

There are important reasons for some prohibitions against the movement of some goods. When Britain banned the export of grains after the English Civil War, for example, it was to keep people from starving. Of course, the crown didn't care if people starved; it just recognized that starving people were more likely to revolt.

Or type the words *orchid* and *smuggling* into Google, and you'll see article after article about how smuggling is one of the major threats to critically endangered species of orchids. The same is true for cacti, succulents, and many other plants. The same is true for many species of animals, from reptiles and amphibians smuggled for the pet trade to elephants killed to smuggle their ivory—to tigers, pangolins, and rhinos killed and smuggled because some fucking assholes think consuming them will make their dicks hard.

So far as I'm concerned, anyone who participates in any of these forms of smuggling can also get in line for their nine-gram ration of lead.

It's okay for communities or institutions of any size or type—from families to towns, to schools, to hospitals, to prisons, to indigenous nations, to nation-states—to prohibit movement of certain goods, or people treated as goods, that harm communities, including the land.

I guess that brings us to at least my own preliminary answer to the morality or immorality of smuggling. The important question is not for me whether something is legal or illegal, promoted or prohibited, but whether it's good for those involved. Good not as in profitable or money-losing, but good as in it makes them healthier and more beautiful.

Armed with this understanding, I spoke with a long-time grower named Fred, who also used to work as a prison guard. Our conversation took place over a half-dozen lunches, separated by a couple of weeks each. I'd gotten an introduction from a mutual friend, Randall, who participated in the conversations.

At one point, Fred said, "I'm glad Randall's here, or I'd have thought you were either winding me up with these questions or making some sort of overtures about trying to smuggle things into prison, instead of just asking about the morality. And honestly, even with Randall here, at first I thought your question was nuts. Nobody who smuggles anything into prison—and I'm with you, in that I was asked a couple of times by inmates and never even considered doing it, but I knew guards who did—thinks about the morality. They're either doing it for money, or if they're visitors bringing it in, doing it for money or for what they think is love.

"But then I thought about your examples of POWs or those in concentration camps, and I think I see what you're getting at. I was able to make up two scenarios in which it could be moral to smuggle drugs into a prison. They're both frankly absurd, and I wouldn't have done it in either case. And both examples involve drugs that are themselves objectively evil. The first is heroin."

Randall interjected, "That shit's nasty. I've had two family members die because of it. They both died years before they finally overdosed. The drug stole them as teenagers, and they passed in their late twenties."

Fred continued, "Oh, I agree. I had a cousin go the same way. I'm just making up a crazy hypothetical. Let's say someone in prison was dying of some horribly painful disease and getting insufficient pain meds. We all know there are some circumstances in which prison medical care is okay, and others where it is . . ." He searched for the word, finally letting the sentence trail off before continuing as though he'd found and said it, "I think one could make the argument that getting him pain relief could be moral."

Neither Randall nor I responded.

Fred said, "So then I really got my teeth into it and tried to make up a circumstance in which it would be moral to smuggle meth into a prison. I hate meth even more than heroin."

I said, "I had several students whose lives had been destroyed by meth."

Randall said, "Don't get me started on what that drug has done to my family as well."

Fred continued, "I was thinking about what you said about concentration camps, and I know that at some slave labor camps they worked people fifteen or twenty hours a day, and if you couldn't hack it, you'd be killed."

I knew where he was going with this, primarily because I knew that although precursors to meth had been used as a decongestant in the early 1930s, use exploded during World War II as soldiers on all sides of the conflict ingested nearly unimaginable quantities of meth. The Japanese alone manufactured and distributed more than a billion pills between 1939 and 1945 to help soldiers stay awake during combat. The results were often miraculous, no matter which soldiers used them. A German field medic wrote in 1942 about a retreat from the Soviets during freezing weather, "In a 14-hour march without contact with the enemy, 25 km were covered in partially deep snow. . . . The snow sometimes being hip-deep, the nervousness (i.e., emotional agitation) of the men resulted in a pace that was too irregular and too rapid. When the ice of Lake Ilmen was reached . . . many comrades showed signs of total exhaustion: staggering, a complete loss of interest and willpower, pain and cramps in the leg muscles, the calves and groin especially, palpitation, pain in the chest, and nausea. Around midnight (6 hours after the retreat had started) some of the troops repeatedly tried to lie down in the snow, their willpower could not be aroused despite vehement encouragement. These men were given 2 pills of Pervitin [meth] each. After half an hour the first men confirmed their improved state of health. They were marching properly again, stayed in line, were more confident and took notice of their surroundings. The pain in the muscles was borne more easily. Some proved to be in a slightly euphoric mood."[10] Euphoric, as they were retreating through hip-deep snow from people who wanted to kill them. Not bad. German tank crews called meth pills "tank chocolates," and air force crews called them "Stuka chocolates," after a type of aircraft. British fighter crews used so many that at least one report stated, "Methedrine won the Battle of Britain." Allied bombing crews—especially tail gunners—routinely took meth to stay awake and alert during long flights.

While meth use may have given soldiers superhuman endurance, it also led to a generation of meth addicts worldwide. It didn't help that through the fifties Japan encouraged meth use among workers to increase productivity, nor did it help that meth was pushed worldwide to help with everything from weight loss to depression cures, to being able to dance all night.

Fred said, "Helping those slave laborers endure—presuming there was an end in sight, otherwise this is just helping the slavers—would, I think, be moral. But other than those two examples, I don't see it, because when we move away from the hypothetical, the truth is that for a lot of prisoners, prison is the first time they've been able to be clean and sober since they were kids or early teens."

I had a minimum-security student named Phil who was extremely concerned about his impending release. He'd been an addict since he was thirteen, and now in his late twenties he was clean, solely and specifically because he was in prison. But, he said, "A condition of my release is that I move back to the county where I offended, which is also the county where I grew up. I can't stay with my mom because she's an addict—where do you think I got my taste for it—and I don't have the strength to watch her use without doing it myself. And I can't stay with my ex-wife because she uses. Our entire courtship, marriage, parenting—hell, our whole relationship—was based on using together. I can't stay with my friends for the same reason. What am I supposed to do, sleep under a bridge?"

---

[10] Unnamed German field medic quoted in Wolfgang U. Eckart, *Man, Medicine, and the State: The Human Body as an Object of Government Sponsored Medical Research in the 20th Century* (Stuttgart: Franz Steiner Verlag, 2006), 69.

And just in the past year I heard from another former student, a nice and smart guy named Kevin who'd been soon due for release from minimum security, where I knew him fifteen or sixteen years ago. He told me he'd gotten out, gone back on drugs, gotten arrested again for theft, then continued his drug use on the inside. The only thing that got him clean was that while in prison he did something stupid—he didn't hint at what it was, nor did I hint at asking—and got sent to solitary for a long stretch. This saved his life, he said, because he couldn't access drugs in solitary. Now, in his late forties—having spent the majority of the previous two decades in prison—he was out, living with his mom and writing a book.

"So here's the thing," I said to Fred and Randall, "Before I taught at the prison, my supervisor told me to always respect my students because 'their punishment is to be removed from society. Their punishment is not to be disrespected by creative writing teachers, or anyone else.' If we were to presume he's right, and that the punitive part is simply to be put in prison, and if for a moment we leave aside rehabilitation, such that prison administrators primarily want to make the institution function as securely, safely, and smoothly as possible, for the public, for guards, for free staff, and for prisoners; then it follows—"

Fred smiled big, wagged his finger at me, then said, "You're a real Sneaky Pete, aren't you?"

"I have no idea what you mean," I responded, only partly truthfully.

"The questions you're really asking," Fred continued, still smiling, "are: 'What are prisons for, and what are drugs for?'"

I didn't say anything.

Fred said, and of course I'm condensing hours of conversation into one exchange, "Whether we believe something is moral is based on whether it aligns with our values. The things that align with our values are, we say, moral. The things that go against our values are, we say, immoral."

"Right," I said tentatively.

He continued, "There are those who don't agree with your supervisor, who think everything about a prison should be as unpleasant as possible, that not only separation from society but existence itself should be punitive. I remember reading that some jail somewhere—I think it was in Idaho—started forcing inmates to use baking soda instead of toothpaste. They did this specifically to make jail even more punishing than it already is. And I worked with a guard who used to delight in withholding toilet paper from prisoners with diarrhea. So, if you want to make prisoners' experiences as bad as possible, deny addicts drugs. Deny them anything that brings pleasure of any sort. Hell, deny them toothpaste and toilet paper. For the punitive-only types, smuggling drugs into prison would be immoral, because it would interfere with the punitive purpose of prison." He paused a moment, then said, "But for enough money probably at least some of them would bring in drugs."

Randall said, "Or toothpaste or toilet paper."

Fred said, "Then there those who believe a primary purpose of prison is rehabilitation. From this perspective, *separating* inmates from drugs would be part of the rehabilitation program."

I told them about Phil and Kevin, and their concerns about relapsing.

"Exactly," Fred responded. "In this case allowing in drugs would be immoral, since it would interfere with the inmates' rehabilitation and would be harming them."

"Yeah," Randall inserted, "And while some people use drugs to expand their minds, we all know that's not why most people use."

I thought about something I wrote in my book *Dreams*: "We can talk all we want about the potential for liberation through . . . ingesting mind-altering substances, but if we're honest, the vast majority of mind-altering substances are not ingested to facilitate better relations between those doing the ingesting and those on other sides (or this side) [in other words, with the cosmos, the divine (however they define that), their muse, their own minds, their family or friends, or nature], but rather to neutralize oppressive reality, to allow those doing the ingesting to either numb themselves out sufficiently to continue to participate in their own degradation under the . . . capitalist system, where everyone and everything (including themselves) has been turned into a commodity; or to vent just enough anxiety . . . to guarantee the pressure of conforming to this system doesn't become so great that people can no longer bear it, and must either break the system or break themselves. Just today, I received an e-mail from someone who wrote, 'Last year I was so overwhelmed by feelings of apathy and depression that I couldn't help myself and started getting back into some bad drug habits. If I can't change anything, I thought, I might as well get drunk/stoned.' The point is that far more drug and alcohol use is actually beneficial to the system of domination . . . than is harmful to . . . [the system] and beneficial to life. It's more a governor that keeps the machine running steadily than it is a sledgehammer used to smash it."

I told Fred and Randall a less flowery, more repetitious, and often incoherent version of this.

Fred responded, "This brings us to those for whom the primary purpose of prison is to warehouse prisoners, those who just want for the institution to run as smoothly as possible. If you leave off the illegality of it, they probably wouldn't mind if some drugs were smuggled in. For that matter, they probably wouldn't mind if drugs were put in the water. Not meth, of course. The last thing you'd want for smooth administration of a prison would be chemically-enhanced paranoia among violent offenders who may very well struggle with PTSD or other mental health issues and who are packed in way too tight with other violent offenders who also may struggle with PTSD or other mental health issues. That would be nuts. But other drugs? Hell, the prison would run very smoothly if everyone was always so stoned they could barely move."

I responded, "From a warehousing perspective, I always thought it would be a good idea to put a computer/playstation in the wall of every cell, and get all the prisoners addicted to computer games. It would be a way for them to kill long stretches of time. There are people who *don't* live in prison who nonetheless voluntarily constrain themselves to a chair in front of a computer to play games for hours every day. And these are people who could be outside, or having sex, or doing *something* besides, as one friend calls it, 'killing pixels.'"

Randall said, "And we all see the connection to the larger society, right? How it's easier to manage a larger society when everyone is drugged?"

I love talking with my friends.

But maybe we were all being unfair. The day we had this part of the conversation, I was suffering a bout of Crohn's disease. In the couple of hours we'd been at the restaurant, I'd had to go to the bathroom six times. My guts were cramping pretty bad. And what would be wrong with alleviating that pain through whatever means necessary? What would be wrong with taking an opiate not only to relieve pain but to slightly constipate me? Many times, Vicodin has helped me get through bouts of Crohn's. And so has marijuana, not by making me so stoned I don't care but by relaxing my spasming guts. And what could be wrong with having given my mother liquid morphine to keep away the pain of the cancer that killed her?

Because I have Crohn's, I've had more than my share of doctors sticking fiber optic cables up my butt to look at the interior walls of my intestines, to see how scarred they are, how many active sores there are, and where the intestines might be blocked. They also have to pump gas into me to inflate my intestines so they can guide the lighted head of the fiber optic cable around my intestines' meanderings. Anesthesia for this process has improved greatly in my life. Early days I was given a nurse's hand to hold and a towel to chew on. Later they gave me a drug that sedated me but kept me awake enough to follow instructions, and also made me forget the procedure once it was over. The first time I was given this, in the recovery room afterwards I made a point of try- ing to remember every step of the process and was fascinated to watch in real time as parts of my memory disappeared, much like details of a dream on awakening. Now they use something even cooler, called propofol, that has as a side effect the stimulation of the brain's pleasure center. I wake up giggling and giddy, and spend the next half hour repeatedly making the same joke with the recovery room nurse about how I want to schedule my next colonoscopy for the following day.

I'll take that over a towel to chew on every time.

And if we ask if it's okay to use substances to numb physical pain, can we not ask if it's okay to also numb emotional pain? When modern Western anesthetics were introduced in the middle of the nineteenth century, many men eschewed their use for such "minor" surgeries as having their teeth pulled or their fingers amputated, because to use them would, they thought, indicate weakness. At this point that seems silly and unnecessary. And aren't we doing something similar now by wanting to feel emotional pain instead of numbing ourselves to it? What's wrong with being comfortable?

And even if you aren't going to numb, what's wrong with just feeling good? Hell, if meth can make you feel slightly euphoric as you're fleeing the Red Army in the middle of winter, give me some of that shit on a normal day and I'll feel like Superman. And pot is known for its ability to adjust your attitude. Cheech and Chong made entire careers out of the fact that stoners will laugh at almost anything. What's wrong with that? And opium poppy seeds were important enough to ancient humans that people were buried with them more than 6,000 years ago. They were cultivated by Sumerians almost 5,500 years ago. Why? Well, the Sumerian name for the plant might give a hint; they called it the "plant of joy." What's wrong with feeling joy, even, or especially, if it comes from a plant?

And if you believe the consumption of mind-altering plant substances is always bad, you'll have to give up your morning tea or coffee, as well as sugar, wheat, and a whole lot of others.

At least some nonhumans consume mind-altering substances. We're all aware of the relationship between cats and catnip. And some dogs and cats like to lick cane toads, who secrete the hallucinogen *bufotoxin*. Vervet monkeys intentionally ingest fermented sugar cane, after which they show decreased coordination and increased socialization. Not having vervet-human dictionaries, scientists have yet to discover if the monkeys are saying, "I love you, monkey. I really do." Capuchins and lemurs disturb poisonous millipedes, then rub them on their bodies, covering themselves with multiple toxic compounds. It is believed they do this to repel insects, but afterwards the capuchins and lemurs enter what looks like "blissful intoxication." Bighorn sheep eat a narcotic lichen—some become so addicted they wear down their teeth scraping it off rocks—and reindeer eat the hallucinogenic *Amanita muscaria*. Reindeer also intentionally drink the urine of humans who have eaten these mushrooms. The mushroom's psychoactive compounds pass relatively unchanged into the urine, suggesting the reindeer are seeking out these compounds, rather than eating the mushrooms for their nutritive value. Rough-toothed dolphins have been observed mouthing highly toxic pufferfish, passing these around like a blunt at a concert, then floating—presumably in more ways than one—motionless and seemingly stoned near the surface. Some people don't believe the dolphins are getting high but rather are becoming temporarily paralyzed by the pufferfish's neurotoxins, but that doesn't explain why they pass the pufferfish around. Wallabies eat opium poppies—Australia provides about half of the world's legally-grown opium, used to make morphine—then jump in circles stoned out of their minds. Water buffalo do the same in illegal fields in Vietnam. Around the world, birds have been known to become drunk on fermented fruits. I've seen this myself, with birds no longer capable of flying and having to ride out the intoxication on the ground. Because this is so common in Australia, they have "Drunken Parrot Season." Post-mortems of dead songbirds in Vienna, Austria, found many of these birds had eaten so much fermented fruit that they'd trashed their livers. Michael Pollan wrote, in *The Botany of Desire*, "Goats, who will try a little bit of anything, probably deserve credit for the discovery of coffee: Abyssinian herders in the tenth century observed that their animals would become particularly frisky after nibbling the shrub's bright red berries. Pigeons spacing out on cannabis seeds (a favorite food of many birds) may have tipped off the ancient Chinese (or Aryans or Scythians) to that plant's special properties. Peruvian legend has it that the puma discovered quinine: Indians observed that sick cats were often restored to health after eating the bark of the cinchona tree."[11] Bears in Kamchatka have been known to become addicted to huffing jet fuel, seeking out the barrels, sniffing, then rolling over on their backs. And jaguars often eat *Banisteriopsis caapi*, one of the primary plants used to brew ayahuasca. It's possible the big cats eat this to cleanse their digestive tracts, which is pretty cool in itself, but afterwards the jaguars are clearly intoxicated. Local

---

[11] Michael Pollan, *The Botany of Desire: A Plant's-Eye View of the World* (New York: Random House, 2001), 117.

indigenous people believe the jaguar consumes the plant to heighten its senses and improve its ability to hunt.

Right now, my elderly kitty has crazy eyes from rolling in the 'nip.

Of course, it's also possible, as an activist working to protect kangaroos told me, that the wallabies aren't trying to get stoned but instead have been forced out of their habitat and are eating food that gets them stoned because there isn't enough other food available to them. She told me that some species of kangaroos will eat grass that is toxic to them, and which causes them to stagger as if drunk, but do so only because their habitat has been so degraded. In extreme conditions humans have been known to eat shoe leather and paper in for the most part vain attempts to stave off starvation. Likewise, it's possible the birds aren't alcoholics, but rather their habitat, too, has been so degraded as to force them to eat inferior food.

We don't really know how often nonhuman animals intentionally ingest mind-altering substances. Some researchers think it happens rarely, and when it does is evolutionarily maladaptive; any creature who gets eaten while stoned will not reproduce, and of course many mind-altering plant substances are themselves toxic. As one analysis puts it, "The use of psychoactive substances [by both humans and nonhumans] can often result in profound detriment to personal health (e.g., cancer, neurodegeneration, liver/kidney/heart failure, overdose, addiction/compulsive drug seeking at expense of self-preservation, etc.) and numerous social ills, which, prima facie, would reduce evolutionary fitness." On the other end of the spectrum are people like Ronald Siegel, who stated, "Almost every species of animal has engaged in the natural pursuit of intoxicants." He believed that the pursuit of intoxication through the use of drugs, alcohol, and psychotropic plants is permanently embedded in the psyche of every human being and that the desire to get high is a drive as strong as that for food, water, and sex.

I honestly don't know.

But here's what I do know.

I know that much has been made over the years of studies showing that if you give rats in a laboratory the choice of pressing a lever to access cocaine or pressing a lever to access food, they'll choose the former, even unto starvation.

But what's less commonly remarked is that other studies show that rats in the wild don't make this same choice. They choose food, and they don't become addicted to cocaine.

I think we all know the implications of this for humans.

I also know that all over the world, drugs, including alcohol, have often been used to subjugate people and to keep them pacified. Pimps have long known this, as prostituted women have been hooked on drugs as long as there has been prostitution, both so the women can numb themselves enough to get through their days, and also so they can't run away.

The Temperance Movement was not, as is commonly portrayed, a bunch of sour-faced old women who wanted to make sure nobody had any fun. Much of it consisted of women who were tired of being beaten by—or seeing other women beaten by—drunk men. In the United States, at least, the Temperance Movement was strongly associated with the Suffrage and the Abolition Movements. And as much as people like to deride Prohibition, it worked: rates of alcoholism dropped, only rising to pre-Prohibition levels in the 1970s. And now? There's a commercial on television proudly proclaiming that Coors is "the official beer of drinking in the shower." I've known precisely one person in my life who needed to drink in the shower, and he was committing suicide by the swallow, taking everyone else in his life down with him.

As early as 1737, American Indians were campaigning against alcohol because of the harms it was causing native peoples. In the nineteenth century, the Lakota Red Cloud laid more blame on alcohol than on weapons for the subjugation of his people. "Friends it has been our misfortune to welcome the white man. We have been deceived. He brought with him some shining things that pleased our eyes; he brought weapons more effective than our own; above all, he brought the spirit water that makes one forget for a time old age, weakness, and sorrow. But I wish to say to you that if you would possess these things for yourselves, you must begin anew and put away the wisdom of your fathers. You must lay up food, and forget the hungry. When your house is built, your storeroom filled, then look around for a neighbor whom you can take at a disadvantage, and seize all that he has! Give away only what you do not want; or rather, do not part with any of your possessions unless in exchange for another's. My countrymen, shall the glittering trinkets of this rich man, his deceitful drink that overcomes the mind, shall these things tempt us to give up our homes, our hunting grounds, and the honorable teaching of our old men? Shall we permit ourselves to be driven to and fro—to be herded like the cattle of the white man?"

Also, I know that earlier, when Fred, Randall, and I said that heroin and meth are evil, we were wrong. Heroin isn't evil. Meth isn't evil. They're just chemicals. No more nor less evil than any other chemicals, from potassium cyanide to dihydrogen monoxide (a.k.a. water), to tetrahydrocannabinol, to sodium chloride, to sucrose. They just are. Good and evil, morality and immorality, inhere in relationships, not objects. It is the relationship of a person to heroin that determines its morality, and it is the relationship of heroin to that person, that person's family, the larger community, to society, and so on. And it is how those relationships affect all of the myriad other relationships within these communities and how a person's relationship to heroin, or meth, or potassium cyanide, or water, or THC, or salt, or sugar affects the person's relationship to him- or herself.

Which doesn't alter the fact that if you ingest potassium cyanide in sufficient quantities, you die, and if you do not ingest dihydrogen monoxide in sufficient quantities, you die.

Heroin to numb the pain of cancer? Sure.

Heroin in an ultimately and inevitably doomed attempt to, as psychiatrist R. D. Laing put it about various self-destructive coping mechanisms, "plug a void plugging a void"? Not so much.

When I was in high school—and sometimes after, though most often as a teen—my mom would gently steer me away from certain people by saying, "You change when you're around him, and I don't like the person you become in those times as much I normally like you."

It usually worked.

Does a person's relationship to meth, heroin, alcohol, or marijuana; or for that matter sugar, wheat, money, sex, or power, make that person better, kinder, truer? Or does it not? Does it make you like yourself better? Does it make those who matter most to you like you better?

When I was a teenager, I realized that morality requires relationship. I came to this understanding, and this may be way too much information, because of masturbation. I was raised a Seventh-Day Adventist, and the church held vigorous debates on the morality of many different actions, from helping the poor (moral) to swearing (immoral), to going to movies (morally acceptable but dangerous, since some said your guardian angel would never enter a movie theater, so for that time you'd be on your own). And they debated the morality of masturbation, with some saying that in the Bible God killed Onan for the sin of, well, Onanism—that is, spilling his seed onto the ground instead of into his wife (whom he inherited from his dead brother, but we'll leave that aside). Therefore, masturbation was a sin (we'll also leave aside that this would technically have been *coitus interruptus* and not masturbation, but Christian theologians from Jerome to Calvin, to the elders of the church to which I adhered as a child have used this as an argument for the sinfulness of masturbation, and interestingly enough, it is this story on which the Catholic Church bases its opposition to contraception). Others argued that because God made our bodies, we should enjoy God's creation. As a teenager I followed this particular debate with fervent and vested interest.

I still remember the slant and texture of moonlight coming in through my window the night I had my realization. I was, er, considering heeding the call of Onan and wondering if this was a sin. Suddenly everything became as clear and clean as the moonlight. If God doesn't exist, I thought, who besides me cares if I masturbate? If God does exist, why would He care? I'm not hurting another, and I'm not hurting myself. I'm not hurting any relationships, and I'm not violating any trusts. In short, no harm, no foul. No harm, no sin. No harm, no immorality.

Full speed ahead.

This story is, of course, generalizable.

I was at Walmart the other day—and we can ask whether Walmart helps or harms individuals, communities, and the planet; certainly, this whole book is about the Walmartization of the marijuana industry—and I saw a walking cadaver. Gray skin, sunken cheeks, sagging eyelids, skeletal frame. Clearly a meth addict. Was his relationship to meth helping him, helping his relationships, helping his community?

I've known people who've said that because marijuana is "the sacred herb," all marijuana growing is by definition good and that all marijuana growing for the last eighty years has been righteous resistance against the unjust war on drugs, the unjust war on this wonderful plant. But what about growers who use rodenticides and in so doing poison not only the mice and rats but also the owls, hawks, bobcats, coyotes, and endangered Humboldt martens who eat them? How are they any better than other ranchers or farmers who poison wildlife? Do the martens feel okay about it because they were killed by people growing pot? And how are marijuana growers who pull water from salmon streams—or other streams, for that matter—any better than almond or alfalfa growers who pull water from the Sacramento River, apple growers who pull water from the Wenatchee, potato farmers who pull water from the Columbia, golf course owners who pull water from the Colorado, or anyone else who dewaters any river?

Not infrequently, big trimming outfits pay women on a tiered scale where the women receive one wage for trimming, a higher wage for trimming topless, and a higher wage still for trimming nude. How is this any less sexist or objectifying than if she weren't working with marijuana but working in any other industry where men pay women to strip?

Growing marijuana, legally or illegally, doesn't grant you papal dispensations for your ecological or social sins.

To believe morality or immorality inheres in the thing itself—marijuana, heroin, sex, money—is to deny the responsibility of the participant by assigning responsibility to the thing itself. Meth or heroin didn't destroy the lives and families of my students. Their own choices did. It wasn't the bullets' fault that my student, Glide, shot two people in a drug deal gone bad, nor was it the drugs' fault.

Sure, many of my students were never given the tools necessary to make good decisions. I had a student who was prostituted by grandparents at the age of five, one who was homeless and on his own by the age of six, many who'd been routinely beaten and/or sexually abused. Why do you think prisoners beat the shit out of pedophiles and other child abusers? It's not an abstract issue to many of them. One told me, "We know why we're in here. We know what started us on the path that put us in prison for the rest of our lives. And we're really angry about it."

But at some point, we're no longer little children in grown up bodies. At some point—having been given the tools or not—we have to make our own decisions.

A friend recently said to me, "I want to tell you about one of the most powerful gifts my mother ever gave to me. It was early one morning, after her boyfriend had yet again beaten her and ransacked our house, broken everything he could get his hands on. Including my mother. She woke me, had me get dressed, then we started walking to the police station. During the walk she was completely honest with me about the mistakes she had made. She said to me time and again, 'You don't have to live this way. You can choose to live differently.' It turns out, healing and choosing differently helps others to get out, too."

So, what's the point? Why did I drag you through all of this? What does morality have to do with marijuana legalization?

Everything.

I know plenty of marijuana wholesalers who sling marijuana but wouldn't sell other drugs because no one has ever overdosed from marijuana. I asked one grower if he's ever concerned that anyone might misuse what he grows.

He said, "I think about that all the time. I don't want teenagers using my pot. We all know the potential harms that come to the brain from too-much-too-early use. And I'm also not thrilled with the idea of anyone burgling houses to get money to support their habit. It's one reason I grow high-end pot: for the most part, my customers are yuppies wanting to chill and stream old movies. Their use isn't going to hurt anyone, including themselves. Am I lying to myself? Maybe. But I do think about it, and I hope any harm caused by use or misuse of my product is counterbalanced by the happiness and/or healing my plants might bring to others."

We all have frameworks on which we base our actions. Codes of conduct, if you will. For some, legality forms the foundation of our code of conduct. If something is legal, it's okay to do. If it isn't legal, it's not okay to do. I think for many this is the default. But if legality isn't the only framework on which you base your actions, some other frameworks will provide that basis. For most within this capitalist system a primary framework is simply, does it make money? This is as true for those who use or claim legality as their framework as it is for those who do not. This is one reason those in power make many of the laws they do: so they or others in power can make money or accumulate power—their primary frameworks—and still follow the framework of legality.

When the local county formed a committee to develop rules for legal marijuana storefronts, someone who owned two of this community's three already-existing, quasi-legal dispensaries volunteered to participate. He owns several buildings in this county. In other words, he's already in the investor class, rather than the working class. When the final rules were released, following state rules on the distance each store must be from a school, and to the point, creating local rules for how far each store must be from any other store—and I honestly think most members of the committee were surprised to realize this after the fact, although I'm guessing this particular member was not—it ends up that the committee had granted this investor a monopoly on storefront space. What a surprise! Every other *possible* storefront location except his own was in a zone of exclusion. The other pre-existing store requested a variance, which the committee denied. Then the committee discovered that one of the monopolist's stores was in fact out of compliance. The committee granted his variance.

Here's the point: with this book I'm merely suggesting that there are other frameworks besides legality and profitability on which to base one's code of conduct. Including morality.

As one grower said to me, "Like most people who've stuck with cannabis, I've had more people than I can count—including the police—rip me off. Because of the liability of opening up to new people, due to 90 percent of people being either incompetent or assholes, I noticed that for many years my interactions have been one-on-one, and that morality was and is an integral component to any relationship within underground business. Any business relationship that has lasted is built around 'I care about you, and we are in this together.'"

Morality underlies the central thesis of this book, that it's better—more moral—to have a decentralized, family- and community-based system of marijuana growing and distribution than it is to have a centralized corporate oligopoly in charge—an oligopoly that would, were it run by underground druglords instead of governments/corporations, be properly called a cartel.

Heck, even if it is run by governments/corporations, the word *cartel*—an association of manufacturers or suppliers with the purpose of maintaining prices at a high level and restricting competition—perfectly describes what marijuana legalization is creating.

The point of this book is that it is not only possible but better—more moral—to have a community-based and human-scale relationship to the cannabis plant.

It doesn't seem right to talk about growing marijuana without discussing pests. If you grow, at some point you're going to encounter them, and you need to be prepared.

Of course, the worst pests in terms of damage to plants, economic harm, and injury to your emotional well-being are humans. They'll sneak into your field or break into your grow room or home, and they'll steal your plants. They'll steal your money. They'll beat your dog. They'll pistol whip or shoot you. They'll sell you pounds that weigh fifteen ounces, and when you sell them seventeen-ounce pounds they'll tell you the pound was short. They'll sell you pot with seeds. They'll steal your change jar. No spider mite or aphid ever stole my change jar.

They'll declare the plant illegal, and when people grow it anyway, they'll put them in prison, and when the public demands the plant be legalized, they'll do so in a way that constitutes a massive transfer of wealth away from family farmers and toward the already-rich. No mold, mildew, or scale ever did that.

I knew a grower who was a few plants over the legal limit. A cop showed up, told the guy he wasn't arresting him but merely overseeing the pulling of the extra plants. So far so good, I guess. Then on the way out, the sheriff made a point of pulling off the driveway and zigzagging his SUV through the grower's vegetable garden.

Humans are the worst pests. Compared to the loss of plants and cash to humans, other pests are trivial.

That said, I have long experience with most types of nonhuman pests.

This should not, however, be perceived as a "how to deal with pests" guide so much as a "how someone who at one time was among the worst growers in the world mostly failed to deal with pests" guide.

First there's the mold *Botrytis*, whom we met earlier. The first step toward getting rid of it was to not grow under the canopy of a temperate rainforest. But when I started growing inside, some plants still got it. The worst part was that because the mold thrives in moist conditions surrounded by lots of sugar, and because air circulates better around or in smaller or larfier buds—buds that are wispy or fluffy—the mold often eats the biggest, tightest buds from inside. You'll have a nice, big, fat cola edging toward maturity when you'll see the tiny leaves that stick out from the cola start to shrivel and change to a color that communicates *Botrytis* to any grower incompetent enough to have seen it as often as I have. You pop open the cola and find a brown, gunky mass growing inside, perhaps similar to what you'd see if you did an autopsy on John Hurt's character in *Alien* with an amorphous chest-burster still inside of him. And then you scream and fall to the ground like Veronica Cartwright's character in that same scene.

Botrytis plagued my plants for a few years until the manager of a grow shop told me how to fix it: use *Cutting Edge Solutions Bulletproof SI* brand silicon dioxide, which was, oddly enough, available in his store for only $77/gallon. He told me the silica—the common name for silicon dioxide—would be taken up by the plants and strengthen their cell walls enough that the mold wouldn't be able to grow into them. I have no idea if his science is accurate or not, and as with so many parts of growing, I don't really care. I just know that it worked. *Botrytis* be gone!

This is a great example of what local communities—including local stores, including family or friendly growers—can provide that eBay/Walmart/Amazon can't. Just as "Recommended for you" at Amazon is no substitute for a conversation with a local bookseller who greets you by name when you enter the store, and who can identify for you "that book with the Irish thing by the female author who wrote that other book where they find a dead body in the hollow of the tree trunk, you know the one, right?"—watching random YouTube videos (including those where a guy wearing a balaclava guarantees you "the dopest method of dealing with mold, man") and buying stuff online is no substitute for asking friendly growers or grow shop owners how to make your, uh, tomatoes grow better.

Long conversations with the grow shop owner—followed by longer conversations with the plants—turned me, for what it's worth, into the grower I am today.

That grow shop went out of business a long time ago. Grow shops don't usually seem to stay in business very long, presumably long enough to launder some money but short enough to not warrant IRS attention. In the last fifteen years six grow shops have come and gone in this tiny town, leaving only one, which I refuse to support. I'll use eBay over supporting that dude. Local community sometimes includes human pests.

Years ago I bought something at a now long-defunct grow shop, then went to the post office, where I left my backpack on a little shelf while I turned to open my PO box. That done, I turned back around, picked up my pack, and went to mail some books.[12] But when I tried to pay, I discovered my wallet wasn't in my pack. I realized immediately I

---

[12] Conveniently available on my website, and I'll sign them for you—and yes, if you ask, I can tell you which one it was where I had the conversation with someone about something or another where we were sitting somewhere and there were pictures of logging on the walls, or something like that. And hey, ain't I great at self-promotion?

must have left it on the counter at the grow shop. I returned, asked the guy if I'd left my wallet, and he smiled and said no. Then I suddenly wondered if at the post office someone had unzipped my backpack and stolen my wallet when my back was turned at the box. That didn't make any sense, but this guy was smiling and telling me no, so what was I to think?

Fast forward a couple of years, and that grow shop had gone out of business, but the same guy happened to be working one day at the shop where I learned so much about growing. I brought a gallon of Grow Big fertilizer to the register, where he charged me eighty bucks. A couple of months later when I needed more Grow Big, the owner happened to be behind the counter. He charged me sixty dollars. I asked him when he dropped his price. He didn't know what I was talking about.

The penny dropped for both of us at the same time.

He asked, "Who was the clerk?"

I knew him well enough to say, "You know who it is, right?"

"That motherfucker." He said his name, which I didn't recognize.

I said, "The guy with the orange hair."

The owner secretly installed a security camera aimed at the register, and caught the guy both overcharging customers and directly stealing from the till.

He's a primary at the town's only remaining grow shop. He's stolen from me twice. I don't need to give him a third chance.

Humans are the worst pests; that guy alone cost me more than *Botrytis* ever did, and no mold ever forced me to cancel my credit card and get a new driver's license.

My plants have also gotten powdery mildew, which expresses as a white powder on the leaves of certain strains. This is a pretty easy one. I just don't grow the strains it likes to grow on.

I've known growers who went apoplectic when people who had powdery mildew in their grow didn't change clothes before coming to visit. Same with *Botrytis*. I've always thought that's silly. I could understand that with certain pests, like aphids, scale, and humans, but spores of powdery mildew and *Botrytis* are both ubiquitous, and unless you've got some biosafety level-four kind of scene going on, you've already got the spores, and they're just waiting for the right conditions. If you've got powdery mildew, either change the conditions, get different strains, or take a couple of hits, because you need to relax, man.

Next are slugs. I like them. Since they eat diseased, dying, or dead leaves, and since their poop is nitrogen rich, I let them roam at will throughout the grow. I've never seen them eat a significant portion of a healthy adult plant. In fact, I think they help control mold by eating dead plant material before it can begin to decompose. I did learn, the hard way of course, to not leave seedlings where slugs can get to them. One morning I walked into the plant room and saw that someone had decapitated all twenty-four of my seedlings. Those seeds averaged $20 each. Attracted to the seedling's tender stems, the slug hadn't touched cuttings the same height. As so often happens, all suffer for the bad behavior of one, so I banished all slugs big and small from the nursery.

I've gotten spider mites a few times. They're fascinating little— less than a millimeter—critters. They, like other arachnids, have eight legs. They're called spider mites not because they're related to spiders (although they are, as well as to ticks and scorpions) but because they sometimes spin webs. They don't spin these webs to capture prey but rather, like tent caterpillars, to protect themselves from predators. Spider mites eat by puncturing plant cell walls and sucking out the innards. Their eggs hatch in three days, and the mites become sexually mature in five. Females lay about twenty eggs/day and live about fifteen to thirty days. So two mites can within a couple of months become somewhere on the order of 300 billion.[13] Even though it would take 150 of them to weigh as much as one stick of gum, their total weight would be about 5,000 pounds, or as much as a midsize automobile. Presuming none of them die.

---

[13] The females can choose whether or not to fertilize each egg, with unfertilized eggs becoming males. Seventy or 80 percent of their young are female. For my rough calculations I presumed two-thirds were female, and the average generation was fifteen days.

Which of course is an unfair presumption, since many would die of old age, and if nothing else, of starvation after they ate all of the plants in the room.

There are four general ways to kill or otherwise get rid of them.

The first is through creating proper conditions for plants to fight off the mites. I don't know if it's a coincidence that ever since I've started feeding the plants silicon dioxide ($77/gallon at the grow shop), I haven't seen many mites. But it's supposed to strengthen their cell walls, and maybe it increases the plants' armor class, so the mites have to roll a seventeen or better on a d20 to strike a hit. Or maybe it's the spiders and other predators I encourage to hang out in the rooms. Or maybe I've just been lucky.

The next is through using neem oil, an organic pesticide made from the oil of the neem tree. It's supposed to be toxic for mites, aphids, and so on, while being safe for birds, mammals (except for humans under some circumstances: for example, pregnant women shouldn't ingest it), and pollinators. It's also moderately toxic for aquatic life. Many growers, including Tim and Mario, swear by it, but either I'm an idiot or for some other reason it was a pain in the ass for me to use, and it never worked for me. I strongly suspect the former.

The next is by using other pesticides. I'm not fond of pesticides, although if they invented one for *Pestis thievus hominus assholonicus* I would use it religiously.

Not only am I not fond of pesticides, I'm not even fond of the word *pest*, except perhaps when applied to the aforementioned *assholonicus*, because honestly most "pests" of agricultural crops are nature trying to repair the wounds that *are* monocrops. If it's true that nature abhors a vacuum, it's equally true that nature loathes a monocrop—which is essentially a vacuum plus one—and will do everything it can to destroy it and return it to its natural state of diversity.

Just right now, standing where forest meets meadow, I can see eight species of trees: coastal redwood, Doug fir, western red cedar, Port Orford cedar, alder, cascara, willow, and a madrone my mom had me transplant from a roadside scheduled for herbicide spraying; at least eight species of bushes: toyon, coyotebrush, huckleberry, salal, thimbleberry, native blackberry, invasive Himalayan blackberry, and invasive cotoneaster; and I have no idea how many species of ferns, grasses, and wildflowers. I can see a dozen types of insects, spiders, birds, and mammals just right now.

Diversity brings resilience, and nature perhaps loves nothing more. A disease striking one species won't kill the whole forest, but only the affected species. And because forests, grasslands, marshes, and others are often mosaics, where one species may predominate in one area and be relatively rare not far away, then common again elsewhere, cataclysmic occurrences like disease may locally extirpate some species, but they can reinhabit from nearby.

There are a few reasons "pests" love monocrops. One is that there are high concentrations of one of their preferred foods in one location; it would be like walking into an unimaginably immense banquet hall—to a spider mite my grow room would be something like six miles long, three wide, and three high—filled with all of your favorite foods.

Plants grown in monocrops have generally been bred to be outlandishly rich in food, fiber (e.g., cotton), or smoke value; and to be defenseless. Bitterness is a defense on the plant's part, as is a harsh smoke, as is toxicity.

It shouldn't be difficult for us to understand these characteristics as plant defense mechanisms. I'm sure most of us know plenty of humans who use bitterness, harshness, and toxicity as defense mechanisms.

So "pests" are presented not only with lots of food, but lots of high quality, tasty, defenseless food.

In nature, predator and prey are by definition generally in balance. Not enough predators and prey increases, leading to abundant food for predators, leading to increased predator numbers, leading to decreased prey numbers. If prey numbers drop too low, predators die, leading to survival of more prey, leading back to more predators. But in a monocrop, predators often have been reduced through destruction of habitat and other means, so in the case of crop pests, not only are the plants abundant, tasty, and defenseless, they also don't have predators to protect them.

This is one reason I encourage and adore the spiders who live in my grow room. I even had some wrentits squeeze through a tiny crack in the wall to roost in there, and I encouraged and adored them as well.

And finally, plants in monocrops aren't in the mosaics we mentioned before, so those who eat them don't have to make long treks through predator-rich inedible plants to start their next feast but can often crawl or fly to the next plant over and continue to gorge. Or they can hitch a ride on your shirtsleeve as you move around your grow room.

All of which is to say I don't consider them pests. I consider them to be just hungry little beings who in nature would be wiping out a monocrop to allow lots of other species to move back in. In fact, from the perspective of the native biome that was replaced by the monocrop—the biome the land wants to bring back—what we call pests could easily be considered instead "pest control," in that they're getting rid of pestiferous plants so the land can get back to doing what it wants and needs to do.

None of which alters the fact that I don't want spider mites to eat all the plants in the room.

And none of which alters the fact that my mother often told me that if I somehow infected her house plants with spider mites, scale, or aphids she would disown me.

I think she was joking, but given how much she loved her house plants, I'm not sure.

When I said I'm not fond of pesticides, I understated. Pesticides, how do I hate thee? Let me count the ways.

One: who was the idiot who came up with the idea of putting poisons on our own food and, just as absurd, putting them on what people inhale into some of the most delicate and receptive tissues in their bodies?

Two: Not content with poisoning ourselves, people and corporations worldwide use more than 5 billion pounds of pesticides per year. Who was the idiot who came up with the idea of bathing the entire planet in nerve agents, endocrine disruptors, and so on? What could possibly go wrong?

Three: Many "pest" insects have short generations, which means they evolve quickly, which means they often evolve resistance quickly. This makes pesticide use ineffective for many of them. Spider mites, for example, are relatively immune to the first several iterations of acaricides people dumped on them. Of course, those with longer generations—humans, for example—would not evolve immunity to these poisons for a very long time.

Four: How long will it take us to learn that it's far easier and safer to work with, rather than against, the world?

Five: Pesticides are just nasty. I remember as a kid being given the task of shooting Raid into a space between boards in the barn where wasps were building a nest. I have no idea why I was supposed to do this; as an adult I've lived near plenty of wasp nests, including one in the mudroom of a home I lived in during my thirties. I made the wasps a deal, told them if they didn't bother me, I wouldn't bother them. The arrangement worked well for both of us. If only I would have had some wasp friends like that a few years later, when the burglars were repeatedly breaking into my home. Maybe I could have somehow sweetened the deal for the wasps: if you sting members of the species *Pestis thievus hominus assholonicus* I'll hook you up with all the rotting peaches you could ever eat. I remember looking at the wasps in the barn when I was a kid, watching them go about their day, and I remember doing what I was told and spraying them, and seeing everyone in the entire nest begin convulsing. I have in the time since killed many thousands of animals and plants—usually either accidentally or to eat—and I've still never been able to forget those wasps. I think of them each time someone talks about poisons.

I even used a pesticide in my grow room once, for an early case of spider mites. I wasn't sure what to do, so I bought a pyrethrin fogger. At least it was natural, made from chrysanthemums.[14] I set it off, and quickly regretted it, because within a second or two all of the spiders in

---

[14] There are some questions about how natural it is. Some of the compounds in it are capable of being synthesized, and in any case the chrysanthemums for it are grown in monocrops. And although it's not particularly toxic to mammals, it's highly toxic to fish and aquatic invertebrates.

the room began to convulse, including any number of mother spiders tending to their babies in their webs.

You could argue that when money's at stake, I should quit worrying about the lives of some spiders up in the corners, but in many ways that's a perfect metaphor for what's wrong with this whole society, with some parts of marijuana culture, and certainly the way marijuana has been legalized. There's something wrong with maximizing revenue at the expense of the smaller ones who live in the corners.

The next method for controlling spider mites is the one I used for several years after the regrettable fogger, which is to introduce predators, in this case predator mites.

Predator mites are, precisely as advertised, carnivorous mites who eat herbivorous mites. You can order them through various insectaries online or by phone. I had enough spider mite problems for a while that I developed a "recognize by voice" relationship with an entomologist at one of the companies. I fear I was less than honest with her, though. She asked what plants the spider mites were eating, and I responded, "My mother loves decorative flowers and houseplants." Literally true, but . . .

Predator mites are grown in hothouses and shipped overnight—the postage is more expensive than the mites—in bags of bean leaves inside a box. You open the box, open the bags, lay the bean leaves on or near the spider mites, do the same with the bags to let out any remaining predators, and let the mites do what animals do: eat. For these suckers—and that's how they eat—this means up to five herbivorous mites or twenty eggs per day. I also bought a species of ladybug called "spider mite destroyers," or *Stethorus punctillum* (who eat up to forty mites per day but are a lot more expensive) and any number of packages of very cheap green lacewing eggs (but never saw a single lacewing larva or adult out of them, so often felt as though I was effectively paying for the rice hulls to which eggs were supposedly attached).

Okay, sperg alert: it pisses me off when even some scientific websites call predator mites cannibals for eating spider mites. *These are scientists*, in some cases entomologists, using this language. But just because they're both mites, doesn't mean they're the same creature. Spider mites and various predator mites share the subclass *Acari*, which encompasses mites and ticks. But they're in different orders (*Trombidiformes* for the former, *Mesostigmata* for the latter). For reference, humans, of the class *Mammalia*, are of the subclass *Theriiformes*, which basically includes all mammals who don't lay eggs, pretty much everyone but echidnas and platypus, and of the order *Primates*. Claims that predatory mites are cannibalistic is the equivalent of claiming that wolves are cannibals because they eat deer, who share their subclass but are in different orders. I'm in awe at both the planet's diversity of life and our near total incapacity or unwillingness to perceive it.

More sperging. Fifteen years ago, I read on one of the insectary websites that not only do predator mites eat spider mites, but they also outbreed them. Because of this I spent a lot of time over the last fifteen years ruminating on why or how it would be in a predator species' best interest to outbreed its prey. I failed to conceptualize any such situation. Perhaps more importantly, I also failed to fact-check that website. Yesterday, just before I was going to write several pages speculating on this extraordinary dynamic, I checked, and no, they don't outbreed their prey. A well-fed predator mite mama might lay two to three eggs per day.

At least I had fun ruminating.

I stopped buying predator mites one year when I couldn't afford them, and found that the mites went away on their own after several weeks. Then for a few years, they would come for a month at the beginning and end of summer. Then they stopped doing even that. I have no idea why.

The next pest I've had lots of experience with is scale, an insect who is really fascinating when they're on someone else's plants. On your own plants, not so much. Let's start by pretending they're on the plants of someone you despise, and talk about how fascinating they are.

Both male and female scale are, on hatching, called "crawlers." They're smaller than a pinhead, and have functioning legs that allow them to crawl to a feeding place, pierce the host plant with a needle-like mouthpart six to eight times the length of their body, and drink its sap.

Some species of scale don't crawl but wait for the wind to blow them to a suitable feeding spot, while others are carried by ants to where the ants keep flocks of them, eating the scales' honeydew—essentially their poop. The crawlers pupate, after which males and females emerge so different that even experts often have trouble identifying them as the same species. Males retain legs, and sometimes wings, resembling gnats. They don't eat, and they live only for two or three days. Their goal is to use their legs or, if available, wings to find a female, which shouldn't be too hard, since a) the ratio of females to males is usually about four to one; and b) females emerge from pupation without legs, remaining unmoving for the rest of their lives. Being plump—by now somewhere between 1/16th and 3/8th of an inch, and so full of sweet liquids that they literally exude it—and immobile is not the optimal defense strategy in a world filled with predators. So the females evolved to exude a waxy armor that more or less seals them to the plant, rendering them impervious to many insect mouthparts as well as many chemicals. Babies are either born live or hatched, depending on the species, under their mother's armor. She will have, again depending on the species, between 400 and several thousand young.

Remember this the next time you're exasperated at having three or four rambunctious children roughhousing inside on a rainy day, and be glad it's not several hundred stuck under your quarter-inch shell.

The first scale probably evolved around 240 million years ago, long before even the first flowering plants. This makes them about six to eight times as old as marijuana, and maybe a thousand times older than humans. They ate the sap of ancient conifers. They survived both the Triassic-Jurassic and Cretaceous-Paleogene extinction events. They're tough. Which is one reason you want them on someone else's plants and not your own.

I asked one master grower how he feels about scale. He thought a moment, then said, "It can be a difficult challenge."

There are a few recommendations I've received for how to deal with this insect. The first is a flamethrower. Any military model should be sufficient. Burn the grow scene to the ground. Burn your house.

Burn your neighbor's house, since that's probably where you got the scale from anyway. Burn all the houses in your neighborhood just to be sure.

And you'll probably still have scale.

The second option is tactical nuclear weapons, or if you have a moral problem with that, call in a predator drone strike with multiple Hellfire missiles. If the missile hits your neighbor's place, presume again that he brought the scale over on his clothes the last time he visited, so your conscience will remain clean.

And you'll probably still have scale.

The third option is to surrender to the obvious wisdom and might of a being a thousand times older than we, flee the country with only what you can carry, hope no scale stowed away on your person or in your clothing, live out your days as a penitent, and pray to whatever gods you believe in that your descendants will not suffer for whatever sins you or your neighbor committed to call scale down upon you.

Make sure you change your name, social security number, and all of your identification cards in a probably vain attempt to keep the scale from tracking and hunting you down.

And you'll probably still have scale.

The next option is to liberally splash rubbing alcohol onto rags and wipe off every leaf and every stem. The rags will become disgusting with scale guts and wax. And you'll miss lots of scale: remember, babies are the size of a pinhead. And scale aren't stupid: they love to grow in tight stem crotches, where it's difficult to get at them. Plan on spending the next several months repeating this process.

And you'll probably still have scale.

You see why my mom threatened to disown me?

I have another dirty rag story. I wear shirts till they fall off my back, socks till the toes can no longer be darned, and underwear till the elastic stretches and the briefs slide under my pants down to my thighs. Then in each case I turn them into rags, which I use till the fabric is so holey as to be nearly beatified, and then I release them to rot in the forest. One time I was feeding molasses to my soil—it feeds the beneficial bacteria and fungi, who spread the joy to the plants—and spilled some on the floor. I grabbed the nearest rag, which happened to be old briefs, and cleaned up the molasses. I walked outside, where I was surprised to see a friend of my neighbor's, some guy in his twenties I'd seen just a few times before. He looked at my face, looked at the brown gooey underwear in my hand, and covered his mouth to abort a retch. "Don't worry," I told him, "It's mine." I took a big lick of molasses, proffered the underwear to him, and said, "It's really sweet. I use it all the time when I bake." He left and never came back.

The next option for dealing with scale is to buy ladybugs. They're cheap, and they and their offspring eat lots of scale. But I hate buying them because they're wild-caught instead of raised in an insectary. Ladybugs overwinter in large clusters, and people harvest them to sell by the thousands. If I knew the ladybugs were invasive—and some species are—then I wouldn't have a problem with this. But if they're native ladybugs—many species of whom are declining—I hate this. Any time you capture any wild being—from insects to birds, to reptiles, to amphibians, to mammals, to plants, to fish, to anyone else for any reason except for very rare captive breeding programs (in other words, when you capture it for pest control, pets, zoos, gardens or hothouses, and so on)—you may as well pulverize it right now, because for ecological purposes the being is dead.

I've agonized over this every time scale has appeared on the plants. Is it worse to buy wild ladybugs, and thus pay to functionally kill thousands of wild beetles from a place I don't know, or to set off a pyrethrin bomb and kill all of the insects and spiders here at home?

Most of the time my answer has been to put off making a decision till the scale have more or less taken over the room, at which time I've finally bought some ladybugs, who in a matter of weeks save the plants from the scale.

It sometimes happens that after the scale are brought under control, the plants have been weakened enough to allow aphids to take hold.

Aphids are even more ancient than scale, having had about 280 million years to perfect their survival strategies, probably the most important of which consists of, like spider mites and scale, having lots of babies really fast. In many species, aphid females can reproduce without males, and to speed things along, these females can be born pregnant. And you thought pregnancy among youth was bad in *your* town.

Aphids have evolved resistance to many categories of pesticide, which leaves us with the same series of options as for spider mites and scale.

Which really brings us to Elisabeth Kübler-Ross. There's a powerful public misconception about Kübler-Ross's important work. Most people believe her articulation of five stages of grief pertained primarily to the death of a loved one. This misperception is reinforced by the titles of her books, like *On Death & Dying*; *On Children and Death*; and *Life Lessons: Two Experts on Death and Dying Teach Us About the Mysteries of Life and Living*. The truth, however—and we can know this by reading her work through the lens of academic postmodern literary theory[15]— is that she came up with her stages of grieving through repeated, long, difficult, and traumatic experiences with aphids.[16]

Denial.

That's not an aphid; it's just a piece of lint.

It was just one aphid. I wiped it off.

I found all the aphids. There weren't that many. No, of course I didn't look on the undersides of leaves. You think I have time for that?

Yeah, there are a lot of aphids, but I think it's going to take care of itself. We just need to ride it out.

Oh my God, this is a lot of aphids, but alcohol rubs/lacewings/lady-bugs/prayers to Jude, the Patron Saint of Lost Causes, will fix it.

---

[15] In other words, by making up the most outlandish horse shit imaginable, then hyperexpanding utilization of unnecessarily obtuse and Brobdingnagian, indeed specious, linguistic/semiotic units and auxiliary obscurational modalities as counterfeit to actual meaning and truth, in the hopes of receiving asspats from other academics whose heads are also so far up their asses that what they think is brilliance is just the fluorescent office lights they see beyond their tonsils: in other words, by making up crap and hoping non-academics are stupid enough to fall for it.

[16] It's a joke! She didn't articulate her stages of grief because of her experiences with aphids! Everyone knows it was because of scale infestations.

Anger.

I'm mad at these damn aphids for killing the plants.

I'm mad at myself for letting the infestation get this bad.

I'm mad at my neighbor, because I just *know* that's where the aphids came from. It couldn't be my fault.

Bargaining.

If you aphids will leave, I'll make a special garden just for you.

If you aphids will let me have just one healthy plant, you can have the rest.

If you aphids will go away at some point in the indefinite future, I will devote my life to the betterment of all aphids, and I will steal and destroy my neighbor's neem oil and pyrethrin bombs.

Depression.

I can't think about the plants anymore without feeling sick to my stomach.

My grow room is no longer a safe space for me; I feel emotionally triggered each time I enter it and need to retreat to a room full of stuffed animals to watch videos of puppies.

There is nothing I can do to defeat the aphid overlords.

Acceptance.

My plants are going to die.

All plants associated with me in the future will die.

My loved ones will die.

I will die.

Aphids will persist.

Eventually the sun will die.

Somehow aphids will find a way to survive this, until in the end only aphids remain.

It is commonly claimed that marijuana—as opposed to alcohol or heroin—has never hurt anyone. I can tell you from direct personal experience this is not true. Marijuana popped my hamstring.

I got tired of the aphids surviving and thriving no matter what I did, so I did the unthinkable: bought a "Doktor Doom" pyrethrin fogger. I caught all the spiders I could find and took them outside, then reached as far as I could over three rows of plants to grasp and tug free the fan's electrical cord (if I kept the fan running, it would blow the poison outside, rendering it useless inside and killing yet more arthropods even farther from ground zero), started the fogger, turned off the lights, shut the door, and left. I came back four hours later, opened the door, turned on the lights, saw far too many dead spiders, felt like a terrible person, walked toward the fan, and picked up the fan's electrical cord, at which time I realized how much easier it is to pull a cord than push it.

The most reasonable solution would have been to take a minute to move the plants out of the way, plug in the fan, return the plants to their original position, and leave.

I'm not always a reasonable person. Holding the plug in my left hand, I extended my right as far as I could, then leaned forward. When I began to tip, I was still six inches from the wall. I leaned even more into it, then toppled till my right hand reached the wall. It worked! Brilliant. I stood on my toes and reached to plug in the fan.

Did I mention that the floor was wet?

My feet started to go out from under me, and in the moment before I threw myself backward, I suddenly remembered that liquids can decrease the coefficient of friction, and remembered also that this coefficient is represented by the Greek letter μ, or mu, which vaguely sounds like a mispronunciation of the first of four syllables I uttered. In the moment after I threw myself backward, I felt a pop in my hamstring.

Marijuana, combined with equal measures of stubbornness and stupidity, popped my hamstring.

It's the least I deserved for setting off a bug bomb.

The remaining spiders were probably cheering.

Oh, and the aphids survived.

If popped hamstrings aren't your thing; if Elisabeth Kübler-Ross isn't your style; and if you happen to live where you can put plants outside; predators, from insects to spiders to birds, will clean your plants faster than you can say, "Nature is your friend."

I was dubious when I learned aphids are an important food source for many bird species. Aphids are tiny—even though there can be a lot of them on an infected plant—so how could this be worth the effort?

I did the math. Let's say a songbird weighs an ounce. There are 28,000 aphids in an ounce, so each aphid would be 1/28,000th of the bird's body weight.

Now, let's say for comparison that I weigh 200 pounds, or about 3,200 ounces. I weigh a bit more than that, but saying 200 makes the math easier and makes me feel better about myself. There are twenty-five potato chips in an ounce, meaning each potato chip is about 1/80,000th of my body weight. Each aphid would be a weight equivalent of a little over three potato chips. Would I bob my head for three potato chips? You bet. Have I already done so? Why do you think there ought to be a + after the 200?

But maybe grapes would be a better comparison, since they, like aphids, are mainly water. There are five grapes in an ounce, or about 1/16,000th of my body weight. So eating an aphid would be for a bird a little over half a grape.

And remember that aphids are full of sweet honeydew. Yum![17]

So now I feel better about the aphid infestation. It's not that I'm a terrible grower; it's that I'm feeding the local wildlife.

---

[17] And yes, I understand that mass isn't what's important. Calories are what's important. But while I may be a nerd, I'm not enough of a nerd to do *those* calculations. . . . Ah, hell, crickets have about 35 calories per ounce—and let's presume aphids are about the same—which compares to about 150 calories per ounce for potato chips and 19 calories per ounce of grapes. To a songbird, an aphid would be the equivalent of about two-thirds of a potato chip or one grape. Still worth it.

CHAPTER 6

History

In the real world, beginnings and endings are never nearly so precise as they are in books.

Think of an individual marijuana plant. When did she begin? When the cutting was made? When the roots started to grow? Or when her mother, grandmother, or great-grandmother began in a seed; or before that when her parents' genes came together in their seeds; or their parents' in theirs?

And when does her story end? At the severing of her trunk? The leaves die slowly, and the roots even more slowly. Are their deaths the end of her story? What about her clone sisters and daughters who still live?

And what about the story of the bud being trimmed, smoked, exhaled, the ash eventually returning to the earth? Does the story end when the THC is in someone's bloodstream, passes the blood-brain barrier, is taken up by cannabinoid receptors in the brain?

I've found that when the juice is too strong, and I start to experience the world in those marijuana-fractured seconds, I sometimes can solve writing or editing problems that had frustrated me for weeks. I don't know if it's because the juice is itself good at writing and editing, or perhaps the juice makes me so stupid and forgetful that I see the writing in a new way. Or maybe the juice sends me down different pathways I wouldn't have thought of without its assistance, makes me see the writing anew, as with the marijuana-induced rapture I felt looking at scallops in peanut butter. And if it does improve my writing and editing, does the story of that plant then extend to you reading what the plant improved?

When molecules of THC, created by and parts of the plant, affect our perceptions and allow us to glimpse the inherent beauty of everything we see, are they helping us to perceive as the plants themselves might perceive, or is it plants and us joining together to perceive this beauty? And when the molecules of THC help us understand that everything we see is in some sense a miracle—from the veins in the backs of our hands to the texture of wet redwood bark, to frog throats full to bursting as they sing, to dogs sleeping deeply on their sides, to bears sleeping that same way—and when the molecules help us see that miracles surround and support us each moment, that we swim through these miracles and that we take them in and let them out with each breath—is this inherent in the THC, or is it a song, a call and response between plant and human, human and plant?

And if the precise beginnings and endings of the stories of individual plants are not always certain, how much more uncertain must be the beginnings of the story of the plant's evolution? Does the story begin with the first life on Earth, or further to the formation of the planet, or further still to the formation of atoms themselves, including the carbon, hydrogen, and oxygen in THC that have made their way from star to rock, to water, to air, to water, to life-form after life-form, to THC, to you?[1]

Or maybe it starts not with the first life, but with the first plants a billion years ago, or the first land plants 470 million years ago (mya), or the first flowering plants from 180 to 130 mya. Or maybe it starts 60 mya, when the family of plants now called *Cannabaceae* diverged from other members of the order *Rosales*.

Cannabis owes its existence, as do elephants, prairie dogs, orangutans, swallowtail butterflies, you, and I, to a big rock. It was between six and nine miles across—some accounts say much bigger—and weighed between a couple quadrillion and a couple of hundred quadrillion pounds. About 66 million years ago, it fell from the sky and landed in a shallow sea near the edge of what is now the Yucatan

---

[1] Yes, I know water is H_2O, with no C, but there's also a lot of dissolved CO_2 in the ocean as well as carbonic acid and bicarbonates.

Peninsula.[2] Its collision with the earth released energy equivalent to a billion Hiroshima and Nagasaki atomic bombs combined, creating a crater more than ninety miles across and twelve to eighteen miles deep. By comparison, the Martian moon *Phobos* is only seven miles across, Mount Everest is less than six miles in elevation and two to three miles above base, the Mariana Trench is less than seven miles deep, and the earth's crust near the Yucatan is six to twenty miles thick.

The impact threw more than 25 million tons of debris into the atmosphere and beyond, making a plume that went halfway to the moon. Tons of this material escaped Earth's gravitational pull, ending up on other planets, in the sun, or in orbit. Other material fell back to Earth, much of it many times hotter than the sun's surface, lighting fire to everything within a thousand miles. As the debris spread, it set most of the world alight: 75 percent of the world's forests burned.

The impact also caused an earthquake a thousand times stronger than any experienced by humans. This, and ensuing underwater landslides, caused tsunamis hundreds of feet tall that covered what would now be several states in the southeastern US, sometimes ripping up rock and soil to depths of hundreds of feet. These waves followed seas, then rivers, all the way to what is now Chicago, and reached Montana with enough remaining power to slam huge fish against trees hard enough to break the fish into parts, then bury them all—fish, trees, rivers—under feet of sediment.

Debris, plus smoke from the fires, turned the sky to night for months, leading to a Narnia-like condition of always winter, never Christmas. Temperatures plummeted.

The collision and ensuing fires had released trillions of tons of greenhouse gases into the atmosphere, so when the dust and ash settled

---

[2] There are some scientists who do not believe the earth was hit with this meteor but that dinosaurs went extinct because volcanoes went hyperactive for tens of thousands of years. If that's the case, you can insert your own dramatic montage leading, no matter the cause, to the extirpation of much life on earth and to a following explosion in speciation as plants, animals, and so on evolved to fill the now-open ecological niches.

many years later, the earth heated rapidly, until both the Arctic and Antarctic were ice free.

Most plants were killed during the ceaseless night. Phytoplankton were mostly wiped out. Between the fire, cooling, heating, and the death of so many plants, 99.99 percent of all living beings died, and 75 percent of all species went extinct. With the exception of some crocodilians and sea turtles, all four-legged creatures larger than fifty-five pounds went extinct.

Some natural communities did okay. Streams, for example, have very little primary production of food by plants. Instead, the food cycle is driven by detritus from the surrounding landscape. And there was certainly lots of that.

It's possible most species of crocodilians survived because they live in rivers, and so were more likely to survive the fires. They're cold-blooded, so can go months without eating; when they do eat, they often scavenge, so for a time they could have feasted. And because their young often eat aquatic invertebrates, who themselves did okay through the cataclysm, this helped ensure the survival of the crocodilian species.

In the oceans, those creatures who directly or indirectly relied on sunlight—phytoplankton, those who ate phytoplankton, and those who ate those who ate phytoplankton—did poorly. By comparison, those living in the deepest parts of the ocean—who mainly scavenged the dead who fell from above or survived off minerals from deep sea vents—did okay.

Back on land, fungi did well, as fungi have done through all mass-extinction events because they, too, primarily eat detritus.

One could easily make the argument that after bacteria, fungi are the most adaptable beings on the planet.

After this near mortal wounding, life did what life does.

Sometimes, the seed of a tree lodges in a tiny crack on a rock face, then germinates. Roots reach for purchase, then food. Water might seep into this crack. The tree grows, until—miracle—you see this tree still clinging to the cliff, somewhere no tree should be able to even survive, much less balance, holding tight to rocks and tighter still to life.

This is life doing what life does.

I once planted a marijuana leaf stem-first in soil, leaf fanning into the air. She sprouted roots. She could not grow into a full plant, since she had no cells to grow stems or flowers, but the leaf grew and grew.

This was life doing what life does.

Many times, I've seen a male bear show off for a female by standing on hind legs facing away from a twenty-foot-tall Doug fir, reaching over his head to grab the trunk in his front paws, then bending forward, pulling down, and breaking the tree over his back. And I've seen those trees continue, either by growing skyward, with some of the highest branches below the break becoming new trunks, or by growing sideways to become bushes, still living after having had their trunks broken.

There's a now-dead tree I dearly love. Long before I moved to this land the tree had fallen, but some of its roots remained in the soil. All of the branches on this tree died, save one, which now, aiming toward the sky, grew into a new trunk. When I first met this tree, the new trunk was forty feet tall. Unfortunately, the new trunk was slightly off-center, and thus slightly out-of-balance, and a few years ago this new trunk fell, rotating the original trunk and yanking the roots from the ground. The tree died. But while it was alive it was life doing what life does.

Now it's being eaten by fungi and is home to mosses. I've seen birds and squirrels rest on it and foxes stand on it, and I've seen claw marks where bears tore at it to get at insects living inside.

So the tree is still life doing what life does.

After the mass extinction—after the initial trauma, the chill, and the fever—life did what life does. Plants reinhabited, and animals followed. But plants had a head-start, as even 1.7 million years later herbivorous insects continued to be relatively rare. It is thought that caterpillars/butterflies/moths evolved at this time to eat and help pollinate plants. The only remaining dinosaurs became in time what we call birds. Mammals, who had diverged from reptiles some 140 million years earlier, but who had both been small and played small ecological roles, evolved to fill more and more ecological niches—or more accurately, *refill*, because until the big rock emptied them, they'd been filled. Reptiles and amphibians did the same. Hell, there were a lot of niches for everyone to fill, and fill they did, till the world ended up home to such miraculous beings as flying, nectar-eating dinosaurs six times the size of bumblebees, with ruby throats and green iridescent heads, who breathe 250 times per minute, tiny hearts beating 20 times per second, tiny wings beating 80 times per second, who can fly 800 miles non-stop, consuming twice their normal fat reserve in doing so, and whose metabolisms are so fast these tiny dinosaurs would starve to death if they did not enter torpor each cold night.

Did you ever wonder how the oceans became so filled with whales? Their ancestors were land carnivores who eventually found that hunting was better underwater, and over the most recent 50 million years evolved into whales, dolphins, and porpoises, including hundred-foot-long, hundred-ton blue whales, whose four hundred-pound hearts beat two to four times per minute, and who eat 80,000 pounds of krill per day (krill weigh about .05 ounces each, so this equates to something on the order of 18 million krill daily).[3]

The point is that a world exuberant and creative enough to evolve nectar-eating dinosaurs whose wings beat far faster than we're capable of seeing as well as basketball-court-length whales with hearts the size of small cars and arteries large enough to comfortably pass basketballs—can also bring into existence a plant scores of millions of years before *Homo sapiens* was even a distant evolutionary twinkle in the eye of *Homo erectus* that, when consumed, can turn peanut butter spoon-scallops into the most beautiful thing I've ever seen.

Isn't that wonderful?

Cannabaceae is a family in the order *Rosales*. Plants in this order are generally woody shrubs to smallish trees, some of whom have thorns. Most but not all have alternate, as opposed to opposite, leaves. Some modern members of this order include roses (of course), strawberries, apples, plums, almonds, elms, figs, mulberries, nettles, and cannabis

---

[3] This would be about 43 million calories per day, or to continue our potato chip comparison from earlier, a little under 18,000 pounds of potato chips, or 28,000 to 35,000 party-size bags.

(also of course). That's not to say these ancient plants necessarily resembled their modern counterparts. Some of these ancestors might have resembled modern wild roses, strawberries, or elms about as much as an ancient *Pakicetus*—a wolf-sized semi-aquatic carnivorous ancestor of cetaceans—resembles a blue whale, or as much as tiny insectivorous early primates resemble you or me.

Nevertheless, there they were, fitting into ecological niches, strengthening their natural communities, and adapting to new circumstances. In other words, speciating, as these natural communities required, requested, forced, caused, created, suggested, or allowed changes in pre-existing species so these species—and the larger communities—would better thrive.

Plants in the family *Cannabaceae* are either upright or climbing, are often sexually dimorphic, and have flowers with no petals and dry, one-seeded fruits. Modern members of this family include some trees, such as hackberries, blue sandalwood, and thorny elms; some vines, such as hops;[4] and some erect herbs, such as cannabis.

There has been a lot of controversy over the *Cannabaceae* designation. In the nineteenth century, cannabis was believed to be in a family only with its closest relative, hops. Then, for a time cannabis was believed to be part of the nettle family, and then the fig family. It wasn't really until a molecular phylogenetic study in 2002 that *Cannabaceae* was again declared to be its own family, but this time with ten genera underneath, including of course *Cannabis* and *Humulus*, or hops. Molecular phylogeny is the study of mainly DNA structures to gain information about some organisms' evolutionary relationships to other organisms. And yes, I had to look that up; and yes, I had to read it several times to understand what it means; and yes, I wish the taxonomical

---

[4] Hops are not technically vines, but bines. Vines use tendrils or suckers to assist in attaching to whatever it is they are climbing, while bines climb by growing in a helix. I would have called them "bines" in the text, but I suspect most of us—myself included—would have thought that was a typo. I love learning new words, and in this case, I thought using the wrong word and then dragging you through this explanation might be a good way for both you and me to remember this distinction. But we'll make it a footnote so that only the adventurous and the pedantic get to learn this great word.

differentiation of cannabis from other plants was as simple as it is for differentiating, say, mammals from reptiles; but no, they're not going to make it that easy for us.

We're not sure when *Humulus* differentiated from *Cannabis*, but it's believed to be between 34 and 6 mya. We know *Cannabis* was here before *Humulus* because fossilized leaves very closely resembling modern cannabis have been dated to 38 mya. For reference, the first great apes began differentiating about 28 mya, the last common ancestor of both chimpanzees and humans lived between 13 and 4 mya, the first members of the *Homo* genus evolved about 2.5 mya, and the first anatomically modern humans lived about 800,000 to 300,000 years ago.

Which means cannabis is definitely older and more than likely wiser than we are.

Before we talk about the history of human relationships with cannabis, we have to talk about endocannabinoid systems, and cannabinoids in general. In other words, what the heck are cannabinoids, what are cannabinoid receptors, why do we have them, and why does this wacky plant produce them?

Most definitions of the word *cannabinoid* are crap. For example, one definition is "any chemical found in cannabis plants." Really? Water is a chemical found in marijuana plants. Is it a cannabinoid? Is lignin—the chemical that makes plant stems woody—a cannabinoid? Of course not. Or "The chemical compounds of cannabis that have an effect on the human body when the plant is consumed." Same deal: water has an effect on me when I consume it, and if I ate enough lignin the fiber would give me diarrhea. Those definitions provide false positives for noncannabinoids. Or, "the narcotic chemicals in cannabis." That definition fails by providing false negatives for the cannabinoids that are not narcotic, which is defined as "a drug that dulls the senses, relieves pain, and brings on sleep."

I shared that one with a doctor friend who advocates for medical cannabis, who responded, "I wish narcotic wasn't such a difficult term for so many for whom it basically equals opiate. When I talk about the effects of cannabinoids, I usually use the words intoxicating, energizing, sedating."

Here's a slightly better definition: "any of a group of closely related compounds which include cannabinol and the active constituents of cannabis." And another: "one of a class of diverse chemical compounds that acts on cannabinoid receptors, which are part of the endocannabinoid system found in cells that alter neurotransmitter release in the brain" and elsewhere.

I shared that last with a chemist friend, who responded, "No good, in my opinion, as this would include structurally unrelated 'cannabinoid-analogues.' I would suggest, 'Any of a group of closely related terpenoid [built from isopentyl-units] compounds which include THC, CBD, and CBN."

So maybe I—and clearly the people who write these definitions on the internet—are going about this backwards. Maybe to understand cannabinoids we should first try to understand cannabinoid receptors, and maybe to understand cannabinoid receptors we should try to understand endocannabinoid systems.

I tried. I searched a bunch of medical and scientific websites for articles on endocannabinoid systems. I didn't have much luck. Oh, there were plenty of articles, some even not behind paywalls, but the articles went way over my head—and I hadn't even been sampling Grandmother Purple. You know things are bad when the only word in the first sentence you've ever seen before, much less know the meaning of, is *lipid*. So, something has something to do with something-something fats, I guess.

So I asked a couple of friends, one of whom is a doctor and longtime advocate for medical marijuana, "What the heck is a cannabinoid system?"

The doctor, Diane Dickinson, said, "It's probably the largest receptor system in our bodies, reportedly larger than our insulin and adrenaline receptor systems. It's involved in every part of our physiology, every organ. A lot of patients—and doctors, too—ask how one plant can help migraines, cancer, depression, psoriasis, and so many other problems, and the answer is that it's because the cannabinoid receptor system is pretty much everywhere.

"I like to start with the history. Cannabinoids were identified by a scientist in the 1930s, but he wasn't able to isolate them. So we knew they existed, but that's about it. Then around 1960, the Israeli biochemist Raphael Mechoulam decided to tackle the mystery of what's in cannabis. At that point cannabis was highly illegal in Israel, so his first problem was how to get some pot to study. He took the direct route— went to the police station, and told them what he wanted to do. They handed him five kilos of hash. He didn't have a car, so he had to take it on the bus-ride home. Everybody on the bus was looking around going, 'What's that smell?'

"By 1963, he had not only isolated CBD, he had determined the molecular structure and synthesized it.

"He tested on monkeys, which is an awful thing to do. In any case, every time they thought they'd isolated a new compound, they'd feed it to the monkeys and see what happened. Time after time there was no detectible response. In 1964 he did the same thing with THC, and all the monkeys went to sleep. So they knew they had something.

"Not a lot of progress was made until 1988, when a team of scientists added a radio tag to THC so it would show up in an x-ray, then injected this into a rat, which of course is also an awful thing to do. They thought the x-ray would show the whole rat light up, but it was all in the brain. They did the experiment again, this time on a human volunteer, and got the same result. This led the scientists to believe there were receptors for THC in the brain.

"When they put out this information to the scientific community, one of the responses was, 'This can't be true, because humans would never evolve a receptor for a plant molecule!' But that's not the right way to look at it. Remember, we make endorphins that are opiates, that are taken up by opioid receptors in the body, which is why opiates made from extracts from opium poppies work after surgery. So the next response was, 'Well, if our bodies can make opiates, maybe they can make cannabinoids. Let's go look.'

"Raphael Mechoulam found the first cannabinoid about two years later. He named it anandamide, since *ananda* is Sanskrit for 'bliss.'

"At this point we know of six cannabinoids that our bodies make. There are probably more.

"The endocannabinoid system got its name because the people who discovered it were studying cannabis. The name is completely appropriate, but by being associated with marijuana the name itself has contributed to the endocannabinoid system being undertaught in most medical schools. If the receptors had been found by somebody who wasn't researching cannabis, it could have a different name, and maybe we'd know a lot more about the system's roles in our bodies."

"I'm a little confused," I said. "What is a receptor?"

My other friend, Jason Stewart, piped up. He's a polymath who trained in molecular biology at Caltech and worked at a biomedical center in Sweden. He got a PhD in computer science in New Mexico and taught high school biology in India. Now he writes plays in Wales. Like I said, a polymath. He answered, "Cells in different parts of our bodies need to communicate with each other. To do that they send chemical messages in the blood, which get carried around the entire body. Eventually the chemicals reach many, many different cells, some being the intended recipients of this or that message and some not. Some messages are general (like when you get frightened by something—say an angry dog running at you—and your body sends out adrenaline as a message) and the message gets accepted by many different cells with different consequences for each different organ or cell type. And some messages are specific, and only one organ, or cell type in that organ, can accept the message.

"The way a cell knows that a message arrives is a bit like someone ringing a doorbell: the chemical message that travels around in the blood is the finger looking for a cell that has the correctly-shaped doorbell to push, and the receptor on the surface of the cell is the doorbell. If the chemical is the right shape for the doorbell, then a 'chime' goes off inside the cell, otherwise the chemical continues traveling through the blood looking for a doorbell. Those chemical messages are called ligands, and they're molecules that bind to receptors.

"All receptors are large, complex protein molecules that are made inside the cell, then carried to the cell membrane and anchored on the surface, spanning the cell wall, so the ligand can dock outside and the 'chime' can go off inside. They live there till they get recycled. Some receptors live a short time before being recycled, while others live for weeks or maybe months before recycling.

"Ligands are most often simple molecules, much smaller than the receptor proteins to which they bind. When the ligand binds/docks to the correct receptor it causes a change in shape of the receptor which makes the 'chime' happen inside the cell. The chime most commonly sends a message to the nucleus of the cell where the DNA lives that causes the cells to either increase or decrease the production of certain other protein molecules.

"Each cell in our bodies has millions of receptor molecules for different purposes. Each tissue of each organ has a specific combination of receptors on the surface, which, among other things, can be used as a marker telling us what organ a cell belongs to and what tissue of that organ it belongs to (which helps us determine if a tumor has metastasized from one organ to another).

"The same receptor can appear on many different tissues and have different functions in those tissues: when adrenaline binds to muscle cells it causes one reaction, and when it binds to brain cells it causes a very different reaction."

The night before this conversation, I'd been having severe enough diarrhea from the Crohn's that I nearly had "an accident." I'm sorry if that's too much information, but the truth is that with Crohn's disease, *nearly* having "an accident" is all-too-often the best possible outcome. So right before I went to sleep, I grabbed a capsule with marijuana materials in it, and, er, packed the trunk. I did this just before sleeping because materials in "the trunk" are absorbed quickly and thoroughly into the bloodstream, and I didn't want to get stoned. I just wanted the diarrhea to stop. It worked. I slept through the night without a single near-accident, without even any urgency.

So I asked, "How does this work? How precisely does THC in the brain mean marijuana-fractured seconds, peanut-butter scallops turning into fine art, and sleepiness—and THC or CBD in other organs means fighting cancer—and THC or CBD in my intestines means causing my guts to relax enough for me to get a good night's sleep?"

Diane and Jason spoke at the same time, "We don't—"

Each looked at the other, motioned for the other to go first, then said again at the same time "We don't—"

They stopped again, started again, stopped again, and I felt like I'd fallen into an Alphonse and Gaston routine, "After you, my dear Alphonse!"

Finally, Diane said, "We don't really know."

Jason said, "It's amazing and mysterious, isn't it? It's fills me with wonder and awe: the incredibly rich tapestry of connections between the plant and animal worlds, a tapestry as ancient as plants and animals themselves. At one point, I would have immediately jumped to offering what knowledge I have to try to fill the gaps in understanding. That was how I was trained as a Western biomedical scientist; everything was understandable and explicable, and imprecision wasn't tolerated. Nowadays I try to remember to slow down long enough to admire the beauty before I charge in and explain it all away.

"So I'll proceed cautiously. One thing to consider is how widespread the endocannabinoid system is. Like Diane said, more widespread than the adrenaline system! And while adrenaline has different effects on different organs—some it excites and some it relaxes (you want your brain in high gear, while you want your muscles poised and ready for quick action)—they're all directed toward the common goal of preparing the body for fight or flight. That's seemingly not the case with the endocannabinoid system, which suggests that cell responses are context-dependent, perhaps mediated by the presence of other chemical stimuli in the cells/blood/tissues."

He continued, "How can a ligand have different consequences in different tissues? The first thought is differences in the tissues themselves: the brain is such a different organ than the colon, so molecules like THC will impact a brain in many ways that it can't impact a colon."

He paused and raised one eyebrow. Diane and I looked at each other.

What is it about scientists and puns? My teachers in college loved them. My freshman chemistry professor ended every lecture with a punny mnemonic. I have to admit it worked; forty years later I can't tell you what an anion or a cation is, but I can tell you that the anion is negatively charged and the cat-ion is puss-itive.

He said, "Also, any ligand can bind to multiple receptors, and those receptors are often tissue-specific, so cells in your colon might have a lot of one receptor, while those in your small intestine might have a very different set. Also, each cell type can have a different 'door chime' hooked up inside the cell, so even though it's still CBD binding to the CB2 receptors, a different set of molecules and pathways carry the signal to where it's received. In one cell-type, CBD might cause certain genes to be turned on, and in another it might cause different genes to be turned off.

"But why CBD and THC? And why do they inhibit diarrhea? Good fortune? And remember, lots of plants interact with lots of animals in ways that affect plants and animals in many different ways. The fruit of the othalanga tree will stop your heart, and oleander is so poisonous that if you even eat the honey, it can make you dizzy, weak, nauseated—and if you eat enough, dead. Opium poppies produce something that can induce euphoria and freedom from pain, and if you take enough of it, you will stop breathing. And of course, still other plants are food for us. We have all of these interactions and relationships with all sorts of plants, animals, fungi, bacteria, viruses, and so on. And— how do I say this—if we weren't talking about marijuana we wouldn't be talking about marijuana. Do you see what I'm getting at? If we were talking about anesthetics, we'd be talking about poppies, and if talking about poisons, we might be talking about oleander. But of all the plants out there, it's possible one might have the effects of poppies, another the effects of oleander, another the effects of coca, another the effects of Queen Anne's lace (which has been used for centuries as a contraceptive and abortifacient), and another the effects of marijuana. And if, I don't know, cascara trees (whose bark is used as a laxative) had the effects marijuana has, then you and I would be talking about how wonderful and amazing it is that cascara has these effects.

"The truth," he said, "is that it's all miraculous. Now, so far as Crohn's, if your bowels are inflamed, causing diarrhea, and if packing some cannabis up there stops the body's response, perhaps the CBD or THC caused chimes to sound that either directly reduced the inflammation or reduced the body's overreaction to the inflammation, just like people with arthritis can slow the body's overreaction in the immune system that attacks their joints.

"So, and I'm just going to make what we in the scientific community call a wild-ass guess, because there's a load of CB2 receptors on immune system cells (T-cells, B-cells, and macrophages), perhaps the cannabis has a relaxing effect on your immune system local to your colon, which means these immune system cells are slowed down and have to receive a much higher stimulus in order to react."

Both Jason and Diane started laughing. I didn't get it.

Jason said, "Basically, your immune cells get stoned and can't put together a coordinated attack on your colon because they're all too busy watching the really pretty swirly patterns floating past."

I asked, "How old is the endocannabinoid system?"

Diane answered, "Probably between 360 and 500 million years. It's been found in every animal they've looked at except crustaceans and insects. This includes invertebrates, even ancient organisms like sea squirts."

Which finally answers the question about to whom we can safely feed leftovers from making marijuana butter without couch-locking them: shrimp, crawdads, and grasshoppers.

I asked, "To be explicit, the endocannabinoid system is older than cannabis?"

"Ten or fifteen times older."

"Which means I and a lot of other people have been thinking about this backwards. I've always thought, as did those scientists you mentioned earlier, that it's extraordinary and miraculous we evolved receptors that respond to chemicals in this plant. But that's not it at all, is it? Instead, it's extraordinary and miraculous that the plant evolved chemicals for which we have receptors."

They both nodded.

And suddenly I understood Diane's point about the endocannabinoid system being understudied because of its name. The endocannabinoid system has nothing to do with cannabis. It existed long before cannabis, in fact it existed 200–400 million years before flowering plants of any kind evolved. It's a hugely important system in the bodies of members of all but two subphyla of animals, with functions we scarcely understand. I said this to Diane and Jason.

Diane responded, "That's true. Raphael Mechoulam said, 'Two eminent scientists at the NIH published that the endocannabinoid system is involved in essentially all human disease. This is a very strong statement, but it seems to be correct. Today we know that the endocannabinoid system—the receptors, the endocannabinoids, the enzymes that form and break down the endocannabinoids—are involved in many physiological reactions, and therefore in many disease states.'[5] The endocannabinoid system is also involved in many healthy states, like pregnancy: If a woman doesn't have cannabinoid receptors in her uterus, embryos can't implant. Your liver has loads of cannabinoid receptors. Your lymphatic system. Your immune system. Your skin. Heck, cannabinoid receptors are important to recovery from head injuries."

None of us said anything for a moment.

Diane broke the silence: "It's a miraculous system, and it's a miracle that this plant interacts with it."

We have a pretty good idea how THC affects our brains, how it: causes munchies, makes us feel good, fractures seconds, interferes with hand-eye coordination, interferes with short-term-something-or-another-I-can't remember-right now.

Endocannabinoid receptors in our brains are especially concentrated in the parts responsible for pleasure, thinking, memory,

---

[5] Raphael Mechoulam, "Raphael Mechoulam and the history of cannabis research," interview by Meir Bialer, *Epigraph* 21, no. 1 (Winter 2019), International League Against Epilepsy, accessed October 28, 2021, https://www.ilae.org/journals/epigraph/epigraph-vol-21-issue-1-winter-2019/raphael-mechoulam-and-the-history-of-cannabis-research.

coordination, and the perception of time. They're located on neurons and are normally activated by the neurotransmitter/ligand anandamide, whom we've already met. Anandamide is made by our bodies and is responsible for mood improvement; appetite regulation; pain management; the creation of short-term connections between neurons; and the facilitation of forgetfulness, which is crucial to maintaining concentration. Imagine how difficult it would be to focus if you were constantly aware of every detail of everything you'd ever perceived or thought.

When THC binds with the receptors in the neurons, it interferes with their communication, which translates to altered perception, experience, and thinking on your part. It can improve your mood, make you feel hungry, reduce your experience of pain, make minutes last for years, and make it impossible for you to remember why you just walked into the living room with a pencil sharpener in one hand and an orange in the other.

All of which still leaves the question: why did cannabis evolve to make cannabinoids?

There are several theories.

The first is the least scientifically-accepted. It's that cannabis evolved these chemicals because God loves us—or if you prefer, nature loves us—or if you prefer, evolution is a mighty and wondrous thing. Is it such a hard stretch to believe that life—which has created such extravagant wonders as the delicate and tender trunk of the elephant, the gaudy beauty of the Vogelkop superb bird-of-paradise's dance, the stalwart heart of the blue whale, the seductive and deadly smell of the pitcher plant, the Santa-Claus-legend-creating power of *Amanita muscaria* mushrooms, and the marvelous wonder-working of those ancestors of retroviruses probably responsible for shaping human intelligence—could also create a plant that makes you feel calm, relaxed, and happy, albeit with the downside of making you think, even if only for a short time, that Cheech and Chong are funny?

Nature is nothing if not miraculous and strange.

Or, if you prefer, God is nothing if not miraculous and strange. Marijuana and Christianity may seem an odd marriage, since a lot of Christian denominations at least nominally oppose drug use—I was raised Seventh-Day Adventist, and using marijuana was considered a Very Big Sin; then again so were dancing and going to movies—but I've known many Christians who've quoted Genesis 1:29, "I have given you every herb-bearing seed which is upon the face of the earth," as they sparked up a fat one, sitting on a couch below their velvet painting of Jesus, Elvis, and Bob Marley sharing a spliff, followed by them singing their favorite hymn: "Jesus loves me, this I know, for the ganja tells me so. All the buds to him belong, some are weak and some are strong."

I bought my first lights from one such Christian. He somehow interspersed quotes from the Bible with his hand-typed directions for the lights. One of the biggest regrets of my adult life is that I didn't save those directions, so I could share with you how he folded the words of Jeremiah into instructions on how to hang a ballast.

Do an internet search for the words "Jesus" and "cannabis," and you will find article after article with headlines like "Experts Now Certain the Key Ingredient in Jesus Christ's Anointing Oil was Cannabis," "Jesus Healed Using Cannabis," and "Was Jesus a Stoner?" This latter article states, and don't blame me for the stoner logic, "If cannabis was one of the main ingredients of the ancient anointing oil, and receiving this oil is what made Jesus the Christ and his followers Christians, then persecuting those who use cannabis could be considered anti-Christ."

The Jesus argument is based on a recipe for anointing oil from *Exodus* that references the herb *q'anah-bosm*, better known as *keneh-bosm*, with the stoners claiming *keneh* means *hemp* and *bosm* means *aromatic*. They also argue that Jesus learned about cannabis when he went to India—although if the recipe is in *Exodus*, he wouldn't have had to leave home—and argue as well that when the Bible describes Jesus casting out demons, he was in fact using cannabis to cure epilepsy and Parkinson's disease.

Jesus and the cannabis area even connected in law. In 2007, the US Supreme Court ruled in what is formally known as Morse v. Frederick, yet is more commonly known as the Bong Hits 4 Jesus case, that high school students do not have the right to hold signs advocating sparking one up for Christ, even when not on school grounds.

Jesus may love marijuana, but the Supreme Court doesn't.

So, marijuana evolved cannabinoids because God or Nature loves us.

That's one theory. And while I'm playing it for laughs—admittedly lamely, hoping you've consumed enough Jamaican Dream to make it seem funny—there are some deeper points to be made here.

One is that a lot of traditional indigenous communities have perceived the world as filled with gifts from a benevolent Creator, and it is part of our task on this earth to comprehend and live the proper relationships between ourselves and these various gifts for which we must in any case show and live gratitude. Many traditional indigenous communities use mind-altering plant or fungus substances medicinally, sacramentally, and most often sparingly.

Is there a relationship between the determining of proper relationships and the necessity of showing gratitude and, for example, the Tolowa Indians living here in northern California for at least 12,500 years without destroying the place?

Another is that a lot of the old-school back-to-the-land type growers unironically call marijuana "the sacred herb." I don't hear that language often from the more corporate or bureaucratic weed producers, except as a hip marketing tool.

Is there a difference in land-use practices between those who grow because they love the sacred herb and those who grow because they can make more money with pot than with tomatoes?

A third is that as psychologist Belinda Gore stated in her book, *Ecstatic Body Postures: An Alternative Reality Workbook*, "Without the opportunity to regularly alter our bodies and our consciousness in a religious trance, we experience what [anthropologist] Dr. [Felicitas] Goodman calls 'ecstasy deprivation.' We live in a society devoid of trance as a regular aspect of our spiritual lives. Many of us living in agricultural and urban settings react unconsciously to this absence of bliss and turn to alternative measures for achieving modified ecstasy. The well-documented addictive behavior that is becoming the psychological hallmark of our contemporary culture is evidence of our ecstasy deprivation. We eat too much of foods that are bad for us, exercise compulsively, and use alcohol, drugs, caffeine, nicotine, work, or sex to relieve the gnawing hunger for bliss."[6]

I'm not sure where the commercial growth or recreational consumption of marijuana fits into all this. I just know that we're missing both sacrament and ecstasy in our lives. We evolved to experience them, and we aren't getting what we need. Can we be blamed, then, for thinking that God or Nature or the Creator has given us gifts to be used sacramentally?

Other theories are more commonly accepted in the scientific, if not the Stoners for Jesus, community.

One is that because THC blocks ultraviolet radiation (UV), and marijuana originated at high altitude, marijuana evolved THC to prevent UV from harming the plant. This theory tells us why cannabis might develop some UV-blocking substance, but not why it might develop one that bonds with receptors in the bodies of so many species of animals.

The next is that THC has antibiotic properties. Plants are eaten by bacteria as surely as are animals, fungi, and other bacteria, and plants need to develop ways to repel or kill these bacteria. So THC might be a way for plants to protect themselves. Which still doesn't explain why the plants would develop an antibiotic that has THC's effects on animal bodies.

The final one I know of is that cannabis evolved THC as a defense against creatures larger than bacteria. Not being able to run or bite, although some can certainly scratch, plants have evolved other ways of discouraging those who would eat them, including producing chemicals that make them taste bitter or that kill the consumer. Perhaps THC is supposed to intoxicate animals, to make them feel so uncomfortable they never eat this plant again; or so comfortable and couch-locked they get eaten by predators, and so cannot eat this plant again; or so

---

[6] Belinda Gore, *Ecstatic Body Postures: An Alternative Reality Workbook* (Santa Fe: Bear & Co., 1995), 13.

forgetful they can't remember where the food source was, and so fail to eat this plant again. This of course explains how THC benefits the plant through developing something that affects animals' endocannabinoid systems. This theory would feel even more compelling if insects responded to THC. When it comes to eating plants, insects are by far the source of most of the action. If I were a plant who was going to develop a resistance to being eaten, I'd probably start and maybe even end with resistance to insects.

But what do I know about anything? Marijuana has lasted on this planet nearly two hundred times as long as humans have.

The discussion above can be reproduced asking why opium poppies produce chemicals that bond with animal opioid receptors. And why nicotine, which evolved as an insecticide, alters human minds.

It's not uncommon for different species to form complex relationships. Some species of flowers release pollen only to the matching species of bumblebee, opening at the precise buzz made by those insects. Some ants herd some aphids and scale, protecting them from predators in exchange for honeydew. The Portuguese man o' war is really not a single creature but a community of creatures. Heck, you're not a single creature but a community of creatures: Ninety percent of the cells inside of you don't have your DNA. They're various bacteria who live in you, digest for you, make you well, make you sick, feed you and feed on you, and after you die, eat you. Even our DNA is not all native to us. Retroviruses have inserted themselves into our RNA and DNA—for example, the retrovirus ancestor just mentioned, the one who climbed inside us and modified us to not only pass on its own genes but to eventually develop in us the sort of intelligence we have.

So it's not necessarily a surprise when some particular plant and some particular species—in this case human—develop some particular relationship.

We don't know when the first nonhuman used cannabis for purposes other than nutrition. We do know that insects were probably eating all parts of the plant from the start, and rodents and birds were eating the seeds.

We can presume that, at first, they ate the seeds for their nutritive value; seeds are stored energy, either utilized by the young plant or by whoever eats the seed. Later, it's possible rodents and birds started eating the seeds for their psychogenic effects. We could even make the argument that cannabis produces THC precisely so that these animals will feel good when they ingest it, leading these animals to gather as many of these seeds as possible—and one pollinated female cannabis plant can produce thousands of seeds. Many birds and rodents store food in so many caches they forget where maybe one-fourth of them are, which is frankly a lot better than I could do. So how smart would it be on the plant's part to produce a chemical that not only makes the animals feel good and want to gather more seeds, and not only makes them hungry for more but also makes these animals forget where the seeds were buried? Basically, the plant would be getting these animals to carry the seeds to new places and plant them.[7]

Which is exactly what the plant has been able to get humans to do as well.

That's pretty smart.

I just saw a series of photos of a little mousie who might be providing anecdotal evidence of this theory. The first photo is of the mousie chewing on someone's marijuana plant. So are the second and third photos. The final photo shows the little mousie lying on his back with a smile on his face, sleeping stoned out of his tiny gourd.

We don't know when, where, or why the first ancient human (or prior, humanoid) used it. Nor do we know how. Did they eat the leaves? Not bloody likely, if my taste buds are an indicator. But lots of medicinal herbs taste bad. Hell, lots of vegetables taste bad (e.g.,

---

[7] Some people claim there isn't any THC in seeds, but that's not true. There isn't as much as there is in buds, but recall that even juiced leaves—which have very little THC compared to the buds—still made my walk home take two hundred years.

brussels sprouts). Just thinking about brussels sprouts made me grab some potato chips to get the imagined taste out of my mouth.

Did they smoke it? Why would they smoke a random plant? Maybe because even back then, teenagers did a lot of stupid shit. Maybe they first tried inhaling smoke from switchgrass and got a headache, bluestem and got a headache, oleander and died. Then someone else inhaled smoke from cannabis and, well, we have a winner.

Or maybe there was a brush fire in a patch of wild cannabis, and people downwind later compared experiences, then got a bright idea.

One plausible scenario for how humans started our relationship with cannabis posits that at some point humans gathered cannabis to eat the seeds (in many places cannabis seeds have primarily been perceived as "famine food" to be eaten only when nothing else is available, but in parts of China prior to the domestication of rice and soy beans, cannabis was considered one of the four main "cereals," along with buckwheat and two types of millet), uprooting whole plants in the fall and carrying them home, where they were threshed. Some seeds slipped away, or were thrown with other plant remains on middens—archeology-speak for trash heaps—where they grew the next spring.[8] Cannabis is often called weed for a reason: it's a pioneer species, an annual enjoying full sun and disturbed, nutrient-rich soil, like in a midden. Thus beginning early the plant's use of humans as mules to carry their seeds from place to place to give them good homes.

Soon these humans were using oil from the seeds for cooking and as a base for soap. They also stripped the stems' outer layers and twisted these fibers into thread, twine, rope. They discovered the process of retting, soaking the stems in water until the non-fibrous parts of the plant rotted and floated away, leaving the fiber. They used this fiber to tie up clothing of animal skins and much later to make the clothing itself; hemp has by now been used for thousands of years to make clothing. One of my most treasured possessions is a vest a traditional indigenous Chinese tailor made from hemp for

---

[8] Robert C. Clarke and Mark D. Merlin, *Cannabis Evolution and Ethnobotany* (Berkely: University of California Press, 2013), 99–100.

my mother to give to me. They used it to make fishing nets, birding nets, nets to catch other animals. They ate the seeds to help with pain. In time, they discovered that inhaling smoke from a burning plant reduced the pain more quickly. They also discovered that ingesting the plant possibly made them better hunters by improving their night vision, allowing them to remain immobile—read, couch-locked—for hours without being bored as they waited in ambush; and by giving them "heightened sensitivity to smells, color, sound, and subtle plays of light and shadow."[9]

There have existed groups of hunter-gatherers whose sole cultivated plant is marijuana, causing Carl Sagan to note that "it would be wryly interesting if, in human history, the cultivation of marijuana led generally to the invention of agriculture and thereby to civilization."[10]

There are also those who—and I don't think I agree with either Carl Sagan or those who make this current point—argue that the ingestion of marijuana and the consequent "ecstatic, visionary effects" was more or less the genesis of religion, "psychologically precipitating the invention and interpretation of invisible spirits, both malevolent and benevolent. If so, these early people came to regard the plant as a gift from their ancestors and their gods to be used as a vehicle for transcending to higher planes of consciousness. Essentially, Cannabis would have provided a means by which they could communicate with their deities—an early 'Plant of the Gods.'"[11]

One problem with this theory is that cannabis isn't native to the Americas, and I wouldn't want to argue that humans living in the Americas had no religions.

---

[9] Clarke and Merlin, *Cannabis Evolution*, 899. They are using the work of Carl Sagan, who argued this in his 1977 book *The Dragons of Eden*.

[10] Carl Sagan, *The Dragons of Eden: Speculations on the Evolution of Human Intelligence* (New York: Random House, 1977). Please note that Sagan was talking about "pygmies" of southern Africa, and some scholars suggest cannabis wasn't introduced to the region until European conquest, with others arguing that cannabis was smoked in southern Africa during the Iron Age. They also argue that the first humans in Madagascar brought it with them.

[11] Clarke and Merlin, *Cannabis Evolution*, 43.

*

Not only do we not know when, where, why, or how humans first used cannabis, but there is also controversy as to what is the oldest archeological evidence for cannabis use. I'm looking at a table in an excellent and exhaustive book on human relationships with marijuana called *Cannabis Evolution and Ethnobotany*. The table shows "Selected ancient fiber artifacts through the ages that reportedly include *Cannabis* [italics in the original] (cloth, cordage, paper, and fiber impressions), ordered by decreasing age."[12] The oldest is from the Czech Republic and dates to between 27,000 and 25,000 years ago. It's not plant material itself, but rather the impression left by "plant fiber cordage"—a piece of net, in this case—on pottery. Armed presumably with the information from this table, it has been reported that "a hemp rope dating back to 26,900 BC was found in Czechoslovakia, making it the oldest known object to be associated with marijuana."[13]

But that's not true. First, it wasn't a rope. It wasn't even a net. It was the impression of a net. Second, a few pages after the table the text states that we don't know the net was made of cannabis. It could have been made of flax, nettle, willow, or any number of other plant materials. It could even have been made, as was true for string made by Neanderthals 90,000 years ago, of the inner bark of pine. Then the text states, "If these impressions could be positively identified as those of Cannabis [capitalized in the original] they would be by far the oldest archeological evidence for its antiquity."[14]

Of course, that's true, but it's also true that if materials collected by a Mars rover could be positively identified as cannabis seeds, then these would be evidence that cannabis is on Mars. Or if the Neanderthal string from 90,000 years ago could be positively identified as having

---

[12] Clarke and Merlin, 176.

[13] Bryan Hill, "Legalized Marijuana: Canada Comes Round to the Wisdom of Ages," Ancient Origins.net, October 17, 2018, accessed October 21, 2021, https://www.ancient-origins.net/history/cannabis-journey-through-ages-003084?fb-clid=IwAR2wmZtxxlrRui_mq4DBar2dsRwiKc0c9xcPkmOAGV3zk4Q4Gbe4Y-IMl9ss.

[14] Clarke and Merlin, *Cannabis Evolution*, 182.

been used to tie a bow on a Christmas present, this would be evidence of the oldest known celebration of the birth of Baby Jesus. Or, as we've all heard so many times, "If there's a bustle in your hedgerow, don't be alarmed now; it's just a spring clean for the May Queen."

If you say *if* at the beginning of a sentence, you can say anything you want for the statement's conclusion.

But maybe I need to unclench my sphincter a little, not only because 26,000 years is a long time to hope plant material doesn't rot but also because a lot of archeology, just like a lot of geology, paleontology, and so on consists of extrapolating theories from tiny bits of information. Someone will hypothesize a religion from a fragment of pottery, a cataclysmic geologic event from specks of dust, a ten-ton dinosaur from a splinter of bone, because that's all they've got to work with, and because—unlike in some of the sciences like basic chemistry or mechanistic physics—you can't generally do real-time experiments to test your hypothesis. A chemist can mix two chemicals and see if they go boom, a physicist can drop a rock off the Leaning Tower of Pisa and see if it falls on someone's head, and scientists can give monkeys THC and see if they fall asleep—but archeologists, geologists, and paleontologists can't always get that physical confirmation. Consequently, I always thought some of the geology classes at the Colorado School of Mines, where I got my physics degree, should really have been called GE101: Guessing at Things; GE201: Pulling Theories from Our Asses; GE301: Advanced Assumptions; and GE401: Mystical Theoretical Conjurations.

I guess I really do need an attitude adjustment.

Which might have been what those ancient humans said moments before the first human-cannabis interaction.

The next 20,000 years led to a lot of what are possibly uses of hemp to make strings, cords, ropes, and nets from Japan to Central Asia, to Europe. And then starting 5,000 years ago we have proof, like fragments of hemp rope, hemp threads and bone needles, a hemp funeral shroud, and so on. We start seeing paper made from cannabis, and paintings on cannabis canvas. We start seeing lots of cannabis canvas cloths, from sails to tents, to clothing. In fact, the word *canvas* derives from the word *cannabis*. Cannabis became an important crop for fiber from Korea to France, to all points between and surrounding.

From 2,500 years ago we have residue from burned cannabis found in incense holders. By then, people across Eurasia were ingesting marijuana medicinally, ritually, and possibly—there's that word—recreationally. Sometimes all at the same time. In China it was written, "To take much makes people see demons and throw themselves about like maniacs. But if one takes it over a long period of time one can communicate with the spirits, and one's body becomes light."[15] A fourth-century sect of Taoism had as one of its eight primary deities *Ma Gu*, literally "Auntie Hemp" or "Hemp Lady." This sect was called the "Highest Clarity School of Mao Shan Mountain,"[16] because, well, centuries may come and go, but stoners never change. The *Atharva Veda* in India calls cannabis one of the five sacred plants, saying of these plants, "let them free us from distress."[17] And the Greek historian Herodotus famously wrote of the Scythians (who originated in steppes on the north sides of the Black to Caspian seas, and who often raided into the Middle and Near East and as far west as Macedonia), "They make a booth by fixing in the ground three sticks inclined towards one another, and stretching around them woolen felts which they arrange so as to fit as close as possible: inside the booth a dish is placed upon the ground into which they put a number of red hot stones and then add some hemp seed . . . . Immediately it smokes, and gives out such a vapor as no Grecian vapor-bath can exceed; and the Scythians, delighted, shout for joy."[18] Strabo tells us of the Mysians, a subgroup of Thracians who lived north and west of the Danube and Dniester rivers

---

[15] Joseph Needham and Lu Gwei-djen, *Science and Civilisation in China: Volume 5, Chemistry and Chemical Technology; Part 2, Spagyrical Discovery and Invention: Magisteries of Gold and Immortality* (Cambridge, UK: Cambridge University Press, 1974), 150.

[16] Clarke and Merlin, *Cannabis Evolution*, 528.

[17] *Atharva-Veda Samhita, Book XI*, trans. William Dwight Whitney, in Harvard Oriental Series, vol. 8, no. 15, ed. Charles Rockwell Lanman, rev. ed. (Cambridge, MA: Harvard University, 1905), 642.

[18] Herodotus, *The Histories—Book IV: Melpomene*, trans. George Rawlinson (1858), 8th ed. (New York: Everyman's Library-Alfred A. Knopf, 1997), 332–33.

(some sources say northwestern Turkey), who were, because of their use of the vapors of heated marijuana seeds for spiritual purposes, called "the *Kapnobatai*," with *Kapnobatai* literally meaning "those who walk in the smoke clouds."[19]

Although people "walked in the smoke clouds," they didn't smoke marijuana, or anything else, for that matter, at least in the way we normally think of smoking. They threw seeds and buds into bowls filled with hot rocks,[20] then breathed in the smoke (after which they shouted for joy), and they burned incense and "drank the smoke" as was said of people in ancient India, but it evidently never occurred to anyone in all of Eurasia, Africa, or Oceana to wrap buds in paper, light this contraption on fire, let it hang from the lips, lean against a wall and do a James Dean impression, nor to put some buds in a small bowl attached to a tube, set them alight, suck smoke through the tube and say, "When you have eliminated the impossible, whatever remains, however improbable, must be the truth," which sounds exactly like something one would say after having done just this.

Cigarettes and smoking pipes were invented by natives of the Americas and were unknown elsewhere until Europeans invaded. Once the inventions were brought back to Europe, however, they spread quickly, such that only forty years after Columbus docked, 3,000 miles away someone was busy inventing the hookah.

Of course he was.

There are some who say Mayans, Aztecs, and other natives of the Americas also used cannabis, and some who even claim that ruins of what we think were Mayan pyramids were instead giant fields of pot, but I fear many of those who say this may themselves have walked a bit

---

[19] According to multiple sources, including: Clarke and Merlin, *Cannabis Evolution*, 515; Strabo, *Geographica* 7.3.3, from *The Geography of Strabo: Literally Translated, with Notes in Three Volumes*, trans. William Falconer and Hans Claude Hamilton, (London: George Bell & Sons, 1903); and William A. Emboden Jr., "Ritual Use of Cannabis sativa L: A Historical-Ethnographic Survey," in *Flesh of the Gods: The Ritual Use of Hallucinogens*, ed. Peter T. Furst (New York: Praeger, 1972), 14–36.
[20] According to the fifth-century BCE philosopher Democritus, they also consumed it mixed with wine and myrrh, after which they would laugh. It is probably not a coincidence that Democritus was known as "the laughing philosopher."

too much in the smoke clouds, because, as we already learned, cannabis isn't native to the Americas.

Throughout much of the world where cannabis did exist, it was important enough to many people that they were buried with it. Scythian tombs often contained marijuana seeds. Same with tombs of the Phrygians in what is now Turkey. You may not have heard of the Phrygians, but I'm sure you've heard stories about some of their leaders: Mygdon, who warred with the Amazons; Midas, whose touch turned everything to gold; and Gordias, whose famous Gordian Knot was cut by Alexander the Great. And can't you just see someone who has walked in the smoke clouds staring at this knot; marveling at the complexity of it all; wanting to unravel it but at the same time not wanting to touch it—knowing that there has never been, and never again will be, a knot with this precise form of complexity; seeing in this knot the beauty and wonder of the interrelatedness of all lives and all beings and all time past and future; and trying to articulate this beauty and wonder, only to have the words slip from consciousness in the hundred years it takes for the thought to move from brain to tongue, emerging instead as a slight giggle or perhaps, following the Scythians, a shout of joy? And can't you see someone else arriving, one of those youths so arrogant he thinks he's going to conquer the world or something, and he's so stoned he thinks it might be the funniest fucking thing to whack at this knot with a sword?[21]

Inside a series of burial mounds in the Altai Mountains of Siberia were wooden frame tents, each holding a bronze vessel filled with stones and the remains of cannabis, leading archeologists to believe the dead were given one final experience of being, well, not necessarily stoned but beautiful, before they continued on their journeys.

Many of the Tarim mummies discovered in northwestern China had

---

[21] It's a joke! We don't know if Alexander the Great was stoned when he cut the Gordian Knot. We don't even know if the Gordian Knot existed. We do know that Alex was fond of intoxicants—he once held a drinking contest with his soldiers in which more than forty of them died from alcohol poisoning—and we also know he sampled the customs of places he conquered, so it's quite possible he encountered cannabis at some point.

been buried with sacks of cannabis next to their heads. Archeologists stated, "The marijuana must have been buried with the dead shamans who dreamed of continuing the profession in another world."[22] One tomb, evidently the final resting place of an ancient Bob Marley, contained one and three-quarters pounds of well-preserved marijuana as well as a wooden bowl with traces of marijuana ash.[23] Another tomb contained the body of a man in his mid-thirties who had thirteen three-foot marijuana plants placed diagonally across his chest.

The extraordinary usefulness of hemp (*hemp* is the name many people use for cannabis grown for fiber) quickly made it central to economies across Eurasia. China became known as the "land of mulberry and hemp,"[24] with mulberry grown to feed silkworms and hemp grown for fiber, food, fun, euphoria, fertilizer, and fighting. Silk was the fabric of the wealthy, while hemp was the "textile of the masses,"[25] becoming, along with ramie and kudzu, one of the three most important plant textiles. Hemp was used for string, yarn, rope, clothing, paper, and canvas, both artistic and pragmatic. It was used for the sails and rigging of warships (and others), and to seal the spaces between planks in the hulls. Marco Polo wrote, "They take lime, and hemp chopped small, and they pound it all together, mixed with an oil from a tree. And after they have pounded them well, these three things together, I tell you that it becomes sticky and holds like birdlime. And with this thing they smear their ships, and this is worth quite as much as pitch."[26] Following the ancient wisdom of "If it ain't broke, don't fix it," fishermen in

---

[22] "Perforated skulls provide evidence of craniotomy in ancient China," *China Economic Net*, January 2, 2007, accessed May 3, 2020, http://en.ce.cn/National/culture/200701/26/t20070126_10220745.shtml.

[23] Clarke and Merlin, *Cannabis Evolution*, 519.

[24] Clarke and Merlin, 334; but I could have chosen a half-dozen different sources. This phrase is common.

[25] H. L. Li, "An Archeological and Historical Account of Cannabis in China," *Economic Botany* 28, no. 4 (1974): 437–48, quoted in Clarke and Merlin, 357.

[26] Colin A. Ronan, *The Shorter Science and Civilisation in China: 3: An Abridgement by Colin A. Ronan of Joseph Needham's Original Text* (Cambridge, UK: University of Cambridge Press, 1986), 116.

Southeast Asia to this day pound twists of hemp bark oakum between planks of their wooden boats to keep them from leaking.[27]

The Chinese were evidently early adopters of Hemp for Victory, since hemp was crucial to not only their navies but their armies. During the Warring States Period (475–221 BCE), someone figured out that hemp made stronger longbow and crossbow strings than the bamboo everyone else was using.[28] This gave them a competitive advantage and presumably led to a dreaded Bowstring Gap and consequent Bowstring Race.

Even today, traditional hunters in Southeast Asia prefer hemp for their crossbow strings.[29]

Not only did the ancient Chinese use hemp in their navies and armies, but also in their air forces: the Chinese invented kites and, as seems to always happen with technological innovation, started using them to kill people. The kite itself was usually silk, and the string was either silk or hemp. Armies used kites to determine distance and facilitate troop movement through difficult terrain, to measure wind, and to communicate. Eventually someone came up with the brilliant idea of adding incendiaries and explosives to the kites.

Hemp was integral to catapults, relying as they did on strong ropes. The Sinologist Herbert Franke wrote in his essay, "Siege and Defense in Medieval China, "The ropes must be made from hemp and leather twisted together, because if the weather is fine, leather shrinks and hemp distends, whereas in rainy weather leather tends to become soft and hemp shrinks. A mixture of the two materials therefore will guarantee uniform operation throughout the year."[30] These catapults could launch huge projectiles hundreds of feet. It didn't take long for innovation in killing to make the projectiles flammable. Again, hemp to the rescue, as sometimes the projectiles contained hemp soaked in oil and

---

[27] Clarke and Merlin, *Cannabis Evolution*, 331.

[28] From *Wujing Zongyau (Essentials of the Military Arts)*, completed in 1043 CE, quoted in Clarke and Merlin, 360.

[29] Clarke and Merlin, 360.

[30] Herbert Franke, "Siege and Defense of Towns in Medieval China," in *Chinese Ways in Warfare*, ed. Frank A. Kierman Jr., and John K. Fairbank (Cambridge, MA: Harvard University Press, 1974), 169.

ignited—may as well give the recipients of these flaming gifts a final chance to be one toke over the line. A recipe for a Chinese gas bomb to produce suffocating smoke included "paper, hemp-bark, resin, yellow wax, yellow cinnabar, and charcoal powder."[31]

They'd also lash hemp to the tails of oxen, set them alight, and stampede them toward their enemy.[32] Sometimes the actions of humans make it so I can't wait for our aphid overlords to take over.

I've heard it said that history is the same characters, different costumes. And a lot of these costumes have been made of hemp.

Korea followed the same pattern as China, with hemp used for string, yarn, rope, clothing, sandals, paper, canvas, supporting cloth for lacquer, and of course war kites. Hemp production peaked in the early twentieth century, only collapsing when replaced by fibers made from petrochemicals. Presumably, when the oil age is over, hemp will again become primary, as it was for thousands of years.

Hemp use in Japan probably began almost 20,000 years ago and also followed the same pattern, including military uses such as bowstrings, clothing for elite warriors and martial artists, and living plants as training tools for ninjas: "The student ninja plants a batch of hemp when he begins training and endeavors to leap over it every day. At first this is no challenge, but the hemp grows quickly every day and so does the diligent ninja's jumping ability. By the end of the season, the warrior can clear the 3–4 meters-high hemp."[33] That's a hell of a high jump. Or, given that the high jumping world record is 2.45 meters, perhaps this is either a "how high must you think I am to believe that" jump or some standard "my buds are the size of baseball bats" dicknanigans.

Hemp was important enough to Japan's World War II efforts that post-war occupying forces prohibited its growth.

---

[31] Franke, "Siege," 169.

[32] Clarke and Merlin, *Cannabis Evolution*, 361.

[33] Dave Olson, "Hemp Culture in Japan," *Journal of the International Hemp Association* 4, no. 7 (1997), International Hemp Association, accessed October 26, 2021, http://www.internationalhempassociation.org/jiha/jiha4114.html.

It took a while for cannabis to get humans to transport it to the Middle and Near East, but when they did, the story was the same. Hemp was used to dress the living and the dead, to make ropes used for building temples where the living could worship, and to make bow strings and catapults to turn these hemp-dressed worshipers into hemp-dressed dead.

Cannabis—or rather hashish—also gave us the word *assassin*.

Or maybe it didn't.

I've debated for several days whether to include this story.

Pro: It's a fascinating story that has been told at least since the time of Marco Polo.

Con: It's probably not true.

Deciding Factor: since when has a story being untrue stopped anyone in marijuana-world (or anywhere else, for that matter) from telling it? It hasn't stopped the posters at the Marijuana Passion or Grasscity forums from talking about their impossibly-huge colas, and it hasn't stopped my neighbor from insisting he didn't somehow sneak aphids into my grow room and into my life while I was sleeping. (And no, pot doesn't make you paranoid, why do you ask?)

It hasn't even stopped me from telling fibs in this book. None of the personal anecdotes in this book are true, except possibly those for which the statute of limitations has passed. And even those are phony as a grow shop conversation about tomatoes.

So here we go. Caveat Lector.

In the late eleventh century, someone named Hassan-i Sabbāh founded a religious sect of Islam called Nizari Ismaili, and then a political state. This wasn't your standard religiopolitical state, though, because instead of seizing and defending territory through the use of armies, his state expanded primarily through religious proselytization and the purchasing of castles, and defended itself mainly through spectacular assassinations of political or military leaders threatening to send armies against them. His people were called the *Asāsiyyūn*, or *Ḥashashiyan*, meaning "people faithful to the foundation of Nizari Ismaili."

Asāsiyyūn fighters were called *fida'i*, which means "one who risks his life voluntarily" and comes from the Arabic word for *sacrifice*. The plural is *fidaiyn*, which you may recognize these days as *fedayeen*. These fighters would become experts in espionage and personal combat and might spend years insinuating themselves into positions close to an enemy leader, where they could publicly kill him, usually with a dagger, and then refuse to flee but wait calmly, seemingly welcomingly, to be killed by the dead ruler's bodyguards.

They were patient, deadly, loyal, and fearless. One story has a visiting ruler claiming he could defeat the Asāsiyyūn because his army was ten times larger. The leader of the Asāsiyyūn responded by telling a fida'i to jump off the castle wall to his death. The man did it without hesitation, and the foreign ruler realized that even with his army he could not defeat such a people.

Another story has a ruler who had sent armies against the Asāsiyyūn waking up one morning to find a dagger stuck in the ground next to his bed. A note soon arrived saying, "Did I not wish the Sultan well, that dagger which was stuck into the hard ground would have been planted in his soft breast."[34] The dagger and note bought twenty-five years of peace.

A third story has a Turkish emir slaughtering thousands of Ismailis, then, becoming concerned he might be assassinated, keeping his bodyguards especially close. Unfortunately for him, two of those bodyguards were fidaiyn, and he was soon dead.

This asymmetrical warfare worked for the Asāsiyyūn for about 185 years, until the Mongols couldn't be assassinated or terrorized away, and effectively destroyed their nation.

It's always been interesting to me that the Asāsiyyūn were hated at the time and still have a bloodthirsty reputation—after all, the word *assassin* comes from the name of their sect—but their method of warfare killed far fewer people than the standard use of armies. They never killed indiscriminately and did not massacre civilians. Many of their

---

[34] Bernard Lewis, *The Assassins: A Radical Sect in Islam* (New York: Basic Books, 2003), 58.

victims had already slaughtered Asāsiyyūn civilians. And they didn't even kill that many leaders—certainly less than a couple of hundred in almost two centuries.

That's far fewer casualties than from the razing of even one village, much less a pitched battle between armies. And the casualties were members of the ruling classes, so what's not to like? Even today, how many leaders do you think would order their militaries to invade other countries if it meant they themselves would be stabbed to death within the year? I'd prefer mutually assured destruction of leaders to mutually assured destruction of entire generations of young people and civilians.

I can hear you say, "Cool story, bro, but if I wanted to read a military history of the Middle East in the twelfth-century, that's what I'd do. Show me the hashish!"

Well, everything I've told you so far is true. But there still remains the question of why and how the fidayin were so placid in the face of sure death.

That's where the story probably becomes apocryphal, first told by Marco Polo to an all-too-credulous audience, an audience whose credulity extends till today.

The courage, in this story, begins with hashish. Asāsiyyūn teen males who showed particular bravery and aptitude for martial arts would for years be told that when they die, warriors of their faith go to heaven, which is filled with unending pleasures. This is of course not unique to the Asāsiyyūn: How many young men or women have been convinced to die for their religion by visions of a wondrous heaven, whether that heaven is religious or secular? What was unique, according to this story, is that some of these young men would be drugged with hashish, then while asleep would be taken to a secret stronghold their leader had prepared and caused to resemble descriptions of this heaven. They'd awaken in beautiful gardens surrounded by beautiful young women who would keep the young men stoned on hashish and who would attend to their every sensual and sexual need. In all physical truth, a patriarchal wet dream.

Add interminable guitar solos and bad cinematography, and we'd also be describing more or less every 1970s rockumentary.

The young men would stay there for about five days—which, coincidentally or not, is how long those two-hour rockumentaries also seemed to last—stoned and sexually exhausted, then would be again put to sleep with hashish and snuck home, where for the rest of their lives they'd eagerly await returning on death to the paradise they'd too-briefly experienced.

You can see how such tangible demonstrations might be more compelling than Pat Robertson-style sermons.

But these demonstrations almost undoubtedly didn't happen this way, if at all.

I can't see how everyone associated with the charade would have been able to effectively keep this secret. And when we learn that Marco Polo's description included streams flowing with water, wine, milk, and honey (!), I'll press X to doubt.

Pretty much everyone accepts that the word *assassin* derives from *Asāsiyyūn* but does not derive from the word *hashish*. The connection between the words was, however, made all the way back when the Asāsiyyūn were still assassinating. This was done intentionally by their political enemies based on the fact that the word for people faithful to Nizari Ismaili— *Asāsiyyūn*—sounds a bit like the word for users of hashish—*Hashishin*. In other words, it was done—and this is something we've seen once or twice in human history—to smear political enemies as sex-crazed, murderous drug users.

And the propaganda worked. Many people still believe this story. I did, until I started researching this section a few pages ago.

Hemp has been grown in Europe for at least 3,000 years and has been as important there as it has been everywhere else it has been grown.

Herodotus again: "They have hemp growing in their country [what is now Romania], very much like flax except for thickness and height. In this respect the hemp surpasses flax by far. This grows by itself and

[is] sown, and out of it the Thracians even make clothing very much like linen."[35] Much traditional women's clothing in Romania continued to be made of hemp into the twentieth century.

A Celtic tomb in southern Germany from about 2,500 years ago had the body of a chieftain laid on an ornate bronze couch covered in a thick cushion of "horsehair, hemp, wool, and the fur of badgers."[36] Jump forward a thousand years, and the Merovingian queen Arnegunde was buried under the Saint Denis Basilica in Paris, wearing a silk dress, surrounded by gold and silver, and wrapped in a hemp shroud.[37]

A guild of hemp weavers was established in France long before a guild of linen weavers.[38]

The Vikings grew a lot of hemp but used more than they could grow, and if you've heard of the Vikings, you can probably guess how they got at least some of the rest: through looting in armed raids they made on ships stitched and caulked together with hemp, with mainly woolen (but some hemp) sails and rigging made of strong, waterproof hemp ropes.

Hemp was used for longbows, and it isn't too much to say that the longbow, with its strong, non-stretching, durable hemp string, revolutionized warfare. As one source put it, the Hundred Years War "witnessed the introduction of innovative weapons [e.g., longbows] and strategy that undermined the traditional system of feudal armies dominated by heavily armored, mounted troops. Powerful new longbows, strung with hemp or flax fibers, allowed effective deployment of standing armies in Western Europe for the first time since the era of the Western Roman Empire."[39]

Hemp was important enough to European economies that multiple kingdoms required landowners to grow it. King Christian IV of Denmark forced farmers to provide hemp for his navy, with law

---

[35] Herodotus, *The Histories*, Book 4, chapter 74, section 1, trans. A. D. Godley (New York: Putnam, 1928), 273.

[36] Quoted in Clarke and Merlin, *Cannabis Evolution*, 282.

[37] It's possible it wasn't her, but the fact remains, someone was buried there with treasures and in a hemp shroud.

[38] Françoise de Bonneville, *The Book of Fine Linen* (Paris: Flammarian, 1994), 76.

[39] Clarke and Merlin, *Cannabis Evolution*, 437.

enforcement officers distributing the seed. Yes, sheriffs delivered mari-juana seeds right to their doors. His grandson Christian V declared that every farmer who didn't sow hemp should "be charged and punished as an obstinate and reluctant servant." And Britain's Henry VIII ordered every farmer controlling sixty acres or more to set aside land for hemp, at risk of a fine of 2–3 percent of annual income. A relative of Anne Boleyn—Henry VIII's second wife, who was executed for "treason" (read, Henry was having an affair and wanted to wring out the old wife and ring in the new)[40]—named Wilyam Bulleyn (and yes, I think it's cool that last names often weren't standardized)—wrote, "This worthy noble herbe Hempe, called *Cannabis* in Latten, can not bee wanted in a common wealth, no Shippe can sayle without Hempe, yᵉ sayle clothes, the shroudes, staies, tacles, yarde lines, warps & Cables can not be made. No Plowe, or Carte can be without ropes * [asterisk in the original] halters, trace &c. The Fisher and Fouler muste haue Hempe, to make their nettes. And no Archer can wante his bowe string: and the Malt man for his sackes. With it the belle is rong, to seruice in the Church, with many mo thynges profitable whiche are commonly knowen of euery man, be made of Hempe."[41]

Wars were fought over hemp, and wars were won or lost because of it. In 2006, Queen Elizabeth II said to a Latvian audience about the 1805 Battle of Trafalgar, "British ships at that time were waterproofed with pitch from Riga, rigged with ropes of hemp from Riga, and their masts were of pine from Riga." Just one sailing ship—military or com-mercial—required more than a mile of hemp rope. The German Press Agency reported on her speech, "During the Napoleonic wars, the French attempted to bar Britain's Royal Navy from the Baltic. British admirals organised convoys of up to a thousand ships at a time to ensure the vital hemp got through. And at the battle of Trafalgar British war-ships rigged with Baltic hemp broke the power of the Franco-Spanish

---

[40] Too soon?

[41] Wilyam Bulleyn, *On Boxyng & Neckweed*, Project Gutenberg, accessed May 12, 2020, https://www.gutenberg.org/files/24790/24790-h/nurture.html. He also states that hangmen's nooses were made of hemp, and that the lives of those who steal shall "end in Hempe."

fleet. The victory is often viewed as the most decisive naval battle in history."[42] It led to British control of the North Atlantic that lasted at least through World War II.

It's probably not fair for me to talk so much about military uses of cannabis, for a couple of reasons. The first is that we'd be hard-pressed to find anything that isn't used either as a cause for war or to kill people once the war has started, from paper to petroleum, to pigs, to pepper, to pigeons, to pachyderms, to pooches, to opium. The second is that hemp has been used for almost everything. Heck, it's been used both as a contraceptive and as an aid to conception; in Serbia it was once believed that to prevent conception women should tie knots in their hemp belts and untie these knots when they wanted to conceive. Alternatively, a woman who wanted to conceive could burn a hemp towel that had been used to wash dishes on the Monday after Palm Sunday, then drink the ashes. Or she could untie a hemp rope bundling hemp stalks, then put it in the water she used to bathe.

I said hemp was used for these purposes. I didn't say it worked.

Some nerds, if you recall, do a lot of drugs. Some don't. I didn't/ don't, depending on whether you count me drinking the juice. Nearly all of my teenage nerd friends didn't. I discovered a different perspective on this the summer I was seventeen.

I was accepted into an eight-week National Science Foundation-sponsored summer science training program at the University of Southern California. Nerd heaven. I brought my multisided dice, ready to kick out the jams with some wild and crazy Dungeons and Dragons games. Let the partying begin!

The thirty-three kids were all, present company possibly excluded, really smart. My roommate's middle name—not a nickname but the name his parents gave him at birth—was Einstein. Fortunately, he was far cooler than the name would indicate, although you might not trust

---

[42] "Queen Praises Latvian Hemp's role in Battle of Trafalgar," German Press Agency (Deutsche Presse-Agentur), October 18, 2006.

me to be the judge of that, having brought multi-sided dice to this coeducational summer event where our living arrangements were more or less unsupervised by adults.

Other than intelligence, though, we were a broad mix, nothing like you'd expect from watching movies. One boy was a typical California surfer dude—tall, slender, usually shirtless, whip smart—with sun-bleached hair and a penchant for responding "Hey, wow!" to almost anything you said to him. Another looked like an old-money teen from central casting—or put another way, like a frat boy into whom someone had transplanted a functioning brain. I don't remember his name, but it should have been Reginald. A third, from New Mexico, was a cowboy with turquoise belt buckle and shit-kicker boots to prove it. Another, from Virginia, was let out of juvie to attend. Think *Good Will Hunting*. He showed up with a knife strapped to his leg and a cigarette hanging from his lips. Of the thirty-three, eleven were girls, which was a great ratio in science those days. They, too, were a wild mix. The East Coast girls were hip—I really dug those styles they wore. But I wish they all could have been California girls with blonde hair and summer dresses, carrying dog-eared and underlined copies of Stendhal or Dostoyevsky for light summer reading—their version of my multi-sided dice—casually quoting Kierkegaard in conversation, and with realistic plans to have PhDs in both physics and chemistry by the time they were twenty-five.

Like I said, nerd heaven. Now if I could only work up the nerve to ask one—a specific one—of the California girls if she wanted to take a bus ride all the way across Los Angeles to a Beatles triple feature of *Help!*, *Let it Be*, and *Yellow Submarine,* followed by a long bus ride back. She'd say yes and love that, right?[43]

---

[43] I did work up the nerve, and she did say yes, and she did in fact love at least the first two movies. We skipped the third to go get a deep-dish pizza. First date ever! When the internet became a thing, I looked her up, and she had indeed gotten her multiple degrees from Caltech and MIT and had gone into medical research, including, it ends up, running a vivisection lab. Two paths diverged in a yellow wood, and all that.

All of which leads to the question: what fragrance would you wear to attract a nerd?

One that smells like π.[44]

The summer went about as one would expect with thirty-three nerd boys and girls away from home mostly for the first time. Lots of reading and nerding for most of us; lots of making out for some; lots of full-on sex for a smaller group; drugs for some; rock and roll for everyone except the disco fanatic from Philadelphia who came complete with a baby blue, wide-collared, polyester leisure suit (rock and roll note: I don't know if you can say you had the peak 1970s concert experience unless you witnessed Blue Öyster Cult's light show while standing next to a socially-oblivious, completely-stoned nerd trying to shout an explanation of how lasers work to a drunk normie attempting to tune him out because he just wants to listen to "Don't Fear the Reaper"); and for more than a few, lots of experimentation with explosives. One boy and girl spent the summer smoking marijuana and having sex in various trees around the campus. He blew off the (scientific) experiments he was supposed to do, and finally, in the last week I had a chance to take my dice from their plastic case so he could use them to randomize his fudged data.

Nerds and drugs go together like chili verde and sour cream: not a necessity but certainly an option.

So it shouldn't surprise us that a lot of early scientists spent a lot of their time stoned out of their gourds. The first English language description of the munchies came from Robert Hooke, who also described the law of elasticity, discovered plant cells, was a seventeenth-century advocate for evolution, was one of a cohort of scientists who together came up with the inverse square law of gravitational attraction, and was not infrequently high. (He frequently got high with a little help from his friend and fellow scientist Robert Boyle.) He wrote, in the third person, of his own experiences consuming pot, "It is a certain plant which grows very common in India. . . . Tis call'd, by the *Moors*, *Gange*; by the *Chingalese*, *Comsa*; and by the *Portugals*, *Bangue*. The

---

[44] My thanks to Laura Drezdzon, who graciously allowed me to steal this joke.

Dose of it is about as much as may fill a common Tobacco-Pipe, the Leaves and Seeds being dried first, and pretty finely powdered. This Powder being chewed and swallowed, or washed down, by a small Cup of Water, doth, in a short Time, quite take away the Memory & Understanding; so that the Patient understands not, nor remembereth any Thing that he seeth, heareth, or doth, in that Extasie, but becomes, as it were, a mere Natural, being unable to speak a Word of Sense; yet is he very merry, and laughs, and sings, and speaks Words without any Coherence, not knowing what he saith or doth; yet is he not giddy, or drunk, but walks and dances and sheweth many odd Tricks; after a little Time he falls asleep, and sleepeth very soundly and quietly; and when he wakes, he finds himself mightily refresh'd, and exceeding hungry. And that which troubled his Stomach, or Head, before he took it, is perfectly carried off without leaving any ill Symptom, as Giddyness, Pain in the Head of Stomach, or Defect of Memory of any Thing (besides of what happened) in the Time of its Operation."[45]
Sound familiar?

Writers can easily be considered a species of nerd. Under the Linnean system they'd probably be *Nerdus literati*, with an older subspecies *Nerdus literati papyrus* and a more recent subspecies *Nerdus literati electronicus*. Muse knows both subspecies have put away a lot of marijuana over the centuries. In nineteenth-century Paris, a group of famous nerds even called themselves the Hashish Eaters Club and met once a month to do as advertised.

The club was founded by psychiatrist Jacques-Joseph Moreau, who had ingested hash in the Far East and experienced hallucinations. He, like many psychiatrists, perceived that hallucinations often preceded mental health breakdowns, and so he believed that if he experienced hallucinations without the ensuing breakdown, he could better understand and thus help his patients. But he still had another problem, which was that while he could ingest hash and experience time distortion and

---

[45] Robert Hooke, "An Account of the Plant, call'd Bangue, before the Royal Society, Dec. 18. 1689," from *Philosophical Experiments and Observations of the late Dr. Robert Hooke* (London: Derham, 1726), 210.

MARIJUANA: A LOVE STORY

other hallucinations, by definition he couldn't clearly and accurately observe while hallucinating. His solution was to form this club and invite a bunch of nerds/artists to ingest hash—by which they meant edibles, made then as now by heating buds in butter, in their case to mix it with cinnamon, cloves, nutmeg, pistachio, sugar, orange juice, butter, and cantharides (!), all melted into their coffee—then watch them trip balls.

Members included a significant portion of mid-nineteenth-century France's most famous writers and artists: Victor Hugo; Eugène Delacroix; Honoré de Balzac; Alexandre Dumas; Gérard de Nerval, who had a pet lobster he walked on a leash (history does not record whether he came up with this idea during one of the monthly meetings); Charles Baudelaire; and many others.

Side note: in a high school literature class one of the students asked the teacher if we were going to read any "Ball Sack" or "Dumb-Ass." Mrs. Carlson had taught enough high school to ignore him, but we sophomores—even we who held *The Count of Monte Cristo* as among the best books ever—thought this was the funniest thing we'd heard in school since eighth grade when we'd learned that "you [plural] drive" in German is "ihr fahrt." We spent the rest of the school year coming up with any excuse we could to say "ear fart."

The writers' descriptions of their experiences with hash are worth reading. Balzac said he heard heavenly voices and saw divine paintings. The journalist Théophile Gautier, writing, like Hooke, in the third person, went into more detail: "A few minutes after swallowing some of the preparation, a sudden overwhelming sensation took possession of him. It appeared to him that his body was dissolved, that he had become transparent. He clearly saw in his chest the hashish which he had swallowed, under the form of an emerald, from which a thousand little sparks issued. His eyelashes were lengthened out indefinitely, and rolled like threads of gold around ivory balls, which turned with an inconceivable rapidity. . . . He now and then saw his friends who were round him disfigured—half-men half-plants, some with the wings of the ostrich, which they were constantly shaking. . . . In the air there were millions of butterflies, confusedly luminous, shaking their wings like fans. Gigantic flowers with challices of christal, large peonies upon beds of gold and silver, rose and surrounded him with the cracking sound that accompanies the explosion in the air of fireworks. His hearing acquired new power; it was enormously developed. He heard the noise of colours. Green, red, blue, yellow sounds reached him in waves. A glass thrown down, the creaking of a sofa, a word pronounced low, vibrated and rolled within him like peals of thunder."[46]

All of this sounds terrifying to me. But some people like it.

Moreau stated, "It is ... *really* happiness which is produced by the hashish; and by this I imply an enjoyment entirely moral, and by no means sensual, as we might be induced to suppose. The hashish eater is happy, not like the gourmand or the famished man when satisfying his appetite, but like him who hears tidings which fill him with joy, like the miser counting his treasures, the gambler who is successful at play, or the ambitious man who is intoxicated with success."[47]

I'm not keen on the idea that a miser counting his treasures is more moral than a famished person sating his hunger, and I'm really not keen on the broader body-hating notion that embodied satisfaction is immoral and the fulfillment of ambition is moral, but his point that it makes a person feel happy remains.

Baudelaire was considerably less taken with the drug. He hated it so much he wrote an essay counting the ways. He wrote, and he, like many nineteenth-century writers, never used ten words when he could use a hundred: "At first it is a certain hilarity, absurdly irresistible, which possesses you. These accesses of gaiety, without due cause, of which you are almost ashamed, frequently occur and divide the intervals of stupor, during which you seek in vain to pull yourself together. The simplest words, the most trivial ideas, take on a new and strange physiognomy. You are surprised at yourself for having up to now found them so simple. Incongruous likenesses and correspondences, impossible to foresee, interminable puns, comic sketches, spout eternally from your brain. The demon has encompassed you; it is useless

---

[46] "Wonderful Effects of Hashish," *Cambridge General Advertiser*, December 20, 1848, 4.

[47] "Occasional Notes," *Pall Mall Gazette*, May 19, 1876, 4.

to kick against the pricks of this hilarity, as painful as tickling is! From time to time you laugh to yourself at your stupidity and your madness, and your comrades, if you are with others, laugh also, both at your state and their own; but as they laugh without malice, so you are without resentment."

Fair enough.

He continues, "This gaiety, turn by turn idle or acute, this uneasiness in joy, this insecurity, this indecision, last, as a rule, but a very short time. Soon the meanings of ideas become so vague, the conducting thread which binds your conceptions together becomes so tenuous, that none but your accomplices can understand you. And, again, on this subject and from this point of view, no means of verifying it! Perhaps they only think that they understand you, and the illusion is reciprocal. This frivolity, these bursts of laughter, like explosions, seem like a true mania, or at least like the delusion of a maniac, to every man who is not in the same state as yourself. What is more, prudence and good sense, the regularity of the thoughts of him who witnesses, but has been careful not to intoxicate himself, rejoice you and amuse you as if they were a particular form of dementia."

After going on and on (and on and on) in this vein, he relays a story some stoners might recognize: "At first dazzled by the beauty of his sensations, he had suddenly fallen into fear of them. He had asked himself the question: 'What would become of my intelligence and of my bodily organs if this state' (which he took for a supernatural state) 'went on?' By the power of enlargement which the spiritual eye of the patient possesses, this fear must be an unspeakable torment. 'I was,' he said, 'like a runaway horse galloping towards an abyss, wishing to stop and being unable to do so. Indeed, it was a frightful ride. . . . It is too late, it is too late! I repeated to myself ceaselessly in despair.'"

True confession: I have been there, when the juice has been too strong, wondering, again and again, moment by moment, "Will I never come back? Did I destroy my brain?"

Baudelaire continues with the story, "'When this mood, which seemed to me to last for an infinite time, and which I daresay only occupied a few minutes, changed, when I thought that at last I might dive into the ocean of happiness so dear to Easterns which succeeds this furious phase, I was overwhelmed by a new misfortune; a new anxiety, trivial enough, puerile enough, tumbled upon me. I suddenly remembered that I was invited to dinner, to an evening party of respectable people. I foresaw myself in the midst of a well-behaved and discreet crowd, every one master of himself, where I should be obliged to conceal carefully the state of my mind while under the glare of many lamps. I was fairly certain of success, but at the same time my heart almost gave up at the thought of the efforts of will which it would be necessary to bring into line in order to win. By some accident, I know not what, the words of the Gospel, "Woe unto him by whom offences come!" leapt to the surface of my memory, and in the effort to forget them, in concentrating myself upon forgetting them, I repeated them to myself ceaselessly. My catastrophe, for it was indeed a catastrophe, then took a gigantic shape: despite my weakness, I resolved on vigorous action, and went to consult a chemist, for I did not know the antidotes, and I wished to go with a free and careless spirit to the circle where my duty called me; but on the threshold of the shop a sudden thought seized me, haunted me, forced me to reflect. As I passed I had just seen myself in the looking-glass of a shop-front, and my face had startled me. This paleness, these lips compressed, these starting eyes!—I shall frighten this good fellow, I said to myself, and for what a trifle! Add to that the ridicule which I wished to avoid, the fear of finding people in the shop. But my sudden goodwill towards this unknown apothecary mastered all my other feelings. I imagined to myself this man as being as sensitive as I myself was at this dreadful moment, and as I imagined also that his ear and his soul must, like my own, tremble at the slightest noise, I resolved to go in on tiptoe. "It would be impossible," I said to myself, "to show too much discretion in dealing with a man on whose kindness I am about to intrude." Then I resolved to deaden the sound of my voice, like the noise of my steps. You know it, this hashish voice: grave, deep, guttural; not unlike that of habitual opium-eaters. The result was the exact contrary of my intention; anxious to reassure the chemist, I frightened him. He was in no way acquainted with this illness; had never even heard of it; yet he looked at me with a curiosity strongly mingled with mistrust. Did he take me for a madman, a criminal, or a beggar? Nor the one nor the other, doubtless, but all these absurd ideas ploughed through my brain. I was obliged to explain to him at length (what weariness!) what the hemp sweetmeat was and what purpose it served, ceaselessly repeating to him that there was no danger, that there was, so far as he was concerned, no reason to be alarmed, and that all that I asked was a method of mitigating or neutralising it, frequently insisting upon the sincere disappointment I felt in troubling him. When I had quite finished (I beg you well to understand all the humiliation which these words contained for me) he asked me simply to go away. Such was the reward of my exaggerated thoughtfulness and goodwill. I went to my evening party; I scandalised nobody. No one guessed the superhuman struggles which I had to make to be like other people; but I shall never forget the tortures of an ultra-poetic intoxication constrained by decorum and antagonised by duty.'"[48]

True confession: I, too, have tried to pretend to be "like other people" when inside I'm feeling "ultra-poetic." It happened when I was interviewed for the *Democracy Now* television program. But I like to think my ultra-poeticity wasn't entirely my fault. It was the result of a Very Bad Medicine, an already-scheduled interview I could not cancel, the unexpected appearance of the ankle of a suddenly-dead man, explosive diarrhea, the clouded judgment that seems to come too often in the soul-piercing dark of three thirty in the morning, and altogether too much chocolate.

Let's start with the Very Bad Medicine. In my twenties I was given extremely high doses of prednisone to attempt to treat Crohn's disease. A potential side effect of prednisone is avascular necrosis: bone death from lack of blood. The talus in your ankle has the lowest blood supply of any bone in the human body, and mine were killed. This led to decades of pain, and by 2010 made me, in the highly technical

---

[48] Charles Baudelaire, *The Poem of Hashish*, translated by Aleister Crowley [!], *The Vaults of Erowid*, accessed May 24, 2020, https://erowid.org/culture/characters/baudelaire_charles/baudelaire_charles_poem1.shtml.

language of the orthopedic surgeon Dr. William Bugbee, "walk like a drunken sailor."

Fortunately, Dr. Bugbee had developed a procedure where he replaces the talus, along with parts of other bones, with those of a dead person. In 2010 I got on the list, waiting for a right-sized talus.

Meanwhile, the activist Randall Wallace had pulled in all sorts of favors to get *Democracy Now* to interview me. An ironclad date was set.

I got a call soon before the interview saying an ankle had come in, asking if I could fly down for surgery within a couple of days. I went. After the surgery and the follow-up, I flew home. Promptly, a Crohn's flare started. Not just any flare, but a grade-A, premium, twenty-shits-a-day-and-lucky-if-none-of-those-are-in-my-pants, knife-in-the-guts flare.

A couple of days into the flare, I flew to San Francisco for the interview. Of course, my flight was cancelled and I had to take a van a couple of hours to the next city over to catch the last flight out. I got in late, checked into a hotel. The interview was set to be recorded at six the next morning.

The pain from the surgery was about what you'd expect from having someone take an oscillating saw to parts of your ankle and tibia, replace them with a dead person's, then screw the whole thing together. In other words, pretty bad, but as a friend's father used to say when I was a kid, "better than a poke in the eye with a sharp stick."

The morning of the interview I awoke at about three thirty in significant pain and even more significant diarrhea. I popped a Percocet—opioids constipate, which in most people is a bad thing, but for me it's a feature, not a bug—which didn't seem to help. I didn't know what to do. I couldn't bear the diarrhea and pain in my guts. Then—and you know how sometimes at three thirty in the morning you don't always make the best decisions—I decided to eat some marijuana-infused chocolate truffle—we know how good cannabis is at calming the intestines. But I ate too much. Way too much.

I fell back asleep. The alarm went off around five fifteen, one hour and forty-five minutes after ingestion, which means the marijuana was really kicking in. This was a catastrophe. I had a television interview in forty-five minutes. It's not too much to say, "I was like a runaway horse galloping towards an abyss, wishing to stop and being unable to do so. 'It is too late, it is too late!' I repeated to myself ceaselessly in despair."

I got to the studio. I guess things could possibly have been worse. At least no one's eyelashes lengthened indefinitely and rolled like threads of gold around ivory balls, nobody shook any ostrich wings, and there were no confusedly luminous butterflies. But I was . . . very comfortable.

Surprisingly, the interview went great. When it aired, lots of people complimented me, saying, "Normally you talk too fast in interviews. But you were so thoughtful. I loved how every time she asked a question, you'd think for a long moment before speaking."

I was surprised no one complimented me on being ultra-poetic.[49]

Back to Baudelaire going on interminably—long enough I thought I must be stoned because every minute of reading seemed like ten years—until he writes, "It happens sometimes that the sense of personality disappears, and that the objectivity which is the birthright of Pantheist poets develops itself in you so abnormally that the contemplation of exterior objects makes you forget your own existence and confound yourself with them. Your eye fixes itself upon a tree, bent by the wind into an harmonious curve; in some seconds that which in the brain of a poet would only be a very natural comparison becomes in yours a reality. At first you lend to the tree your passions, your desire, or your melancholy; its creakings and oscillations become yours, and soon you are the tree. In the same way with the bird which hovers in the abyss of azure: at first it represents symbolically your own immortal longing to float above things human; but soon you are the bird itself. Suppose, again, you are seated smoking; your attention will rest a little too long upon the bluish clouds which breathe forth from your pipe;

---

[49] The interview was only part of the reason I couldn't cancel. A bigger part was that Randall Wallace had also created an all-day conference that I was to host, called Earth at Risk, about stopping violence against the earth and against women. Too much time, energy, and money had gone into it to allow me to cancel. The event went fine, although after every presenter I had to scramble to the bathroom, clenching my sphincter tighter than Fred Phelps's in a San Francisco bathhouse.

the idea of a slow, continuous, eternal evaporation will possess itself of your spirit, and you will soon apply this idea to your own thoughts, to your own apparatus of thought. By a singular ambiguity, by a species of transposition or intellectual barter, you feel yourself evaporating, and you will attribute to your pipe, in which you feel yourself crouched and pressed down like the tobacco, the strange faculty of smoking you!

"Luckily [sic], this interminable imagination has only lasted a minute. For a lucid interval, seized with a great effort, has allowed you to look at the clock. But another current of ideas bears you away; it will roll you away for yet another minute in its living whirlwind, and this other minute will be an eternity. For the proportion of time and being are completely disordered by the multitude and intensity of your feelings and ideas. One may say that one lives many times the space of a man's life during a single hour. Are you not, then, like a fantastic novel, but alive instead of being written?"

He writes all of this as though it's a bad thing.

He calls hashish a "raging demon" that causes a "moral ravage . . . so great, a danger so profound, that those who return from the fight but lightly wounded appear to me like heroes escaped from the multiform Proteus, or like Orpheus, conquerors of Hell. You may take, if you will, this form of language for an exaggerated metaphor, but for my part I will affirm that these exciting poisons seem to me not only one of the most terrible and the most sure means which the Spirit of Darkness uses to enlist and enslave wretched humanity, but even one of the most perfect of his avatars."

Baudelaire seems offended that "If you are one of these souls your innate love of form and colour will find from the beginning an immense banquet in the first development of your intoxication. Colours will take an unaccustomed energy and smite themselves within your brain with the intensity of triumph. Delicate, mediocre, or even bad as they may be, the paintings upon the ceilings will clothe themselves with a tremendous life. The coarsest papers which cover the walls of inns will open out like magnificent dioramas. Nymphs with dazzling flesh will look at you with great eyes deeper and more limpid than are the sky and sea. Characters of antiquity, draped in their priestly or soldierly costumes, will, by a single glance, exchange with you most solemn confidences. The snakiness of the lines is a definitely intelligible language where you read the sorrowing and the passion of their souls. Nevertheless, a mysterious but only temporary state of the mind develops itself; the profoundness of life, hedged by its multiple problems, reveals itself entirely in the sight, however natural and trivial it may be, that one has under one's eyes; the first-come object becomes a speaking symbol. Fourier and Swedenborg, one with his analogies, the other with his correspondences, have incarnated themselves in all things vegetable and animal which fall under your glance, and instead of touching by voice they indoctrinate you by form and colour. The understanding of the allegory takes within you proportions unknown to yourself. We shall note in passing that allegory, that so spiritual type of art, which the clumsiness of its painters has accustomed us to despise, but which is really one of the most primitive and natural forms of poetry, regains its divine right in the intelligence which is enlightened by intoxication. Then the hashish spreads itself over all life; as it were, the magic varnish. It colours it with solemn hues and lights up all its profundity; jagged landscapes, fugitive horizons, perspectives of towns whitened by the corpse-like lividity of storm or illumined by the gathered ardours of the sunset; abysses of space, allegorical of the abyss of time; the dance, the gesture or the speech of the actors, should you be in a theatre; the first-come phrase if your eyes fall upon a book; in a word, all things; the universality of beings stands up before you with a new glory unsuspected until then. The grammar, the dry grammar itself, becomes something like a book of 'barbarous names of evocation.' The words rise up again, clothed with flesh and bone; the noun, in its solid majesty; the adjective's transparent robe which clothes and colours it with a shining web; and the verb, archangel of motion which sets swinging the phrase. Music, that other language dear to the idle or the profound souls who seek repose by varying their work, speaks to you of yourself, and recites to you the poem of your life; it incarnates in you, and you swoon away in it. It speaks your passion, not only in a vague, ill-defined manner, as it does in your careless evenings at the opera, but in a substantial and positive manner, each movement of the rhythm marking a movement understood of your soul, each note transforming itself into Word, and the whole poem entering into your brain like a dictionary endowed with life."

Am I a bad person—is there something wrong with me—for thinking this sounds beautiful?

From there Baudelaire marches right over the top, boldly anticipating *Reefer Madness* and "Demon Weed" by nearly a hundred years. Keep in mind as you read the following that Baudelaire tore through the trust fund his parents set up for him, mainly wasting the money on fancy clothes, wine, parties, even more parties, and even more parties that moved the needle far into the "drunken debauch" category. After his father's death he more or less constantly hectored his mother for money, all while defrauding merchants and landlords by skipping out on lines of credit and past-due rent, and all while whining about how alienated and oppressed he was. (Unfortunately, I've known more than a few people like that—inside and outside of marijuana-world—and in some cases I've been one of the people the narcissistic little shits have skipped out on.) He writes, "Since we have seen manifest itself in hashish intoxication a strange goodwill toward men, applied even to strangers, a species of philanthropy made rather of pity than of love (it is here that the first germ of the Satanic spirit which is to develop later in so extraordinary a manner shows itself), but which goes so far as to fear giving pain to any one, one may guess what may happen to the localised sentimentality applied to a beloved person who plays, or has played, an important part in the moral life of the reveler." Yes, he's calling goodwill toward others "the first germ of the Satanic spirit," which I guess is not out of line with what a wastrel and a thief might think.

I'll quote him a few more times. "Shall I explain how, under the dominion of the poison, my man soon makes himself centre of the Universe? how he becomes the living and extravagant expression of the proverb which says that passion refers everything to itself?" And, "They say, and it is nearly true, that this substance does not cause any physical ill; or at least no grave one; but can one affirm that a man incapable of action and fit only for dreaming is really in good health, even when every part of him functions perfectly? Now we know human nature sufficiently well to be assured that a man who can with a spoon-ful of sweetmeat procure for himself incidentally all the treasures of heaven and of earth will never gain the thousandth part of them by working for them." And, "The gambler who has found the means to win with certainty we call cheat; how shall we describe the man who tries to buy with a little small change happiness and genius? It is the infallibility itself of the means which constitutes its immorality; as the supposed infallibility of magic brands it with Satanic stigma. Shall I add that hashish, like all solitary pleasures, renders the individual useless to his fellow creatures and society superfluous to the individual, driving him to ceaseless admiration of himself and dragging him day by day towards the luminous abyss in which he admires his Narcissus face?"[50]

While he has a point that there are lazy narcissistic little shits who use marijuana, and there are those whom marijuana makes lazier, more narcissistic, and shittier, I find it extraordinary—or rather all-too-or-dinary—that a trust-fund dandy who runs up debts and skips out on them has the gall to call other people narcissistic, useless to their fellow creatures, and to accuse them of not working for what they've got.

Well, I guess I'm quite the Mr. Crankypants today, aren't I? I'm not showing much of that "satanic spirit" of "strange goodwill" and "philanthropy" toward Baudelaire.

It seems yet again I'm in profound need of an attitude adjustment.

I'm back, attitude adjusted, and ready to talk about Vikings, who probably brought the first hemp to the Americas in the rigging and caulking of their ships. In addition, recently, scientists have discovered hemp pollen near a Viking settlement in Newfoundland, which sug-gests the possibility Vikings also brought and planted seeds.[51]

If they raised hemp, the plant probably didn't stay in the Americas longer than the Vikings themselves, even though when the Spanish and the rest of the European thieves explorers arrived in the fifteenth

---

[50] Baudelaire, *The Poem of Hashish*.
[51] Owen Jarus, "Were the Vikings Smoking Pot While Exploring Newfoundland?" *Live Science*, July 15, 2019, accessed May 2, 2020, https://www.livescience.com/65940-were-vikings-smoking-pot-in-newfoundland.html.

and sixteenth centuries, they occasionally reported seeing vast fields of it growing wild. For example, French explorer Jacques Cartier wrote, "At last we came to a very fine and pleasant bay. There is a little river here, and a safe harbor. We named this the St. Croix on account of the day we arrived . . . [where] grows a fine hemp as in France without any sowing or cultivation."[52] But Cartier and the others were wrong, either mistaken or more likely making stuff up to get funding for more ~~armed thievery~~ exploration.

Hemp was brought to Mexico by the conquistador Pedro Cuadrado, who marched alongside Hernán Cortés. Cuadrado established a successful hemp growing operation, expanding rapidly until in 1550 he was compelled by the Spanish governor to "limit production because the natives were beginning to use the plants for something other than rope."[53] Take from that what you will.

Soon hemp agriculture spread north into California, and also all the way into South America.

Independently, in 1606 cannabis was introduced into Nova Scotia by Canada's first apothecary, Louis Hebert, who was also Canada's first European farmer.[54]

Because hemp is so easy to grow in a wide variety of temperatures and habitats (it's called *weed* for good reason) it was soon grown extensively throughout the Americas, used for rope, cloth, paper, and so on, much the same as in the rest of the world. Large hemp farms were everywhere from Boston to Santa Barbara, from Newfoundland to Valparaiso.

While it may have been easy to grow, making money at it was not. Both George Washington and Thomas Jefferson tried and failed to make money growing hemp, which is something I now share with the first and third presidents of the United States. Thomas Jefferson wrote,

---

[52] Jacques Cartier, *The Voyages of Jacques Cartier*, originally translated and edited by Henry Percival Biggar, with an introduction by Ramsey Cook (Toronto: University of Toronto Press, 1993), 105.

[53] Ernest Abel, *Marijuana: The First Twelve Thousand Years* (New York: Plenum, 1980), Schaffer Library of Drug Policy, accessed October 28, 2021, https://druglibrary.org/schaffer/hemp/history/first12000/4.htm.

[54] Clarke and Merlin, *Cannabis Evolution*, 319.

"The shirting for our laborers has been an object of some difficulty. Flax is so imperious to our lands, and of so scanty produce, that I have never attempted it. Hemp, on the other hand, is abundantly productive and will grow forever on the same spot. But the breaking and beating it, which has always been done by hand, is so slow, so laborious, and so much complained of by our laborers, that I have given it up."[55]

Growing hemp became more profitable during the Revolutionary War, as demand grew for hemp rope, sail, and paper products. Hemp was so important to the war effort that those involved in the making of rope or sail for even six months were exempt from military service for the war's duration. Because of hemp's importance, and because of a distrust of paper money, hemp became more important than cash as a standard of exchange for the first few decades of the republic.[56]

Cannabis was grown for psychoactive purposes as well, with high THC varieties probably being brought to the Americas—specifically to the West Indies—by indentured laborers from India, who also brought the understanding that unfertilized buds—buds without seeds—make a stronger high.

Now would be the time to put in that famous quote by Thomas Jefferson, "Some of my finest hours have been spent on my back veranda, smoking hemp and observing as far as my eye can see," which might be something a lot of people would now share with the third president of the United States.

The problem is that Thomas Jefferson didn't say this until 2008.

Likewise, much is made of George Washington separating male from female plants, implying he had learned to smoke seedless pot, but while he did in fact separate males from females, so have most people who've ever grown hemp for fiber: male plants are larger and coarser.

So we don't really get to make presidential pot jokes until Clinton, although he, Bush, and Obama are all fair game. All of whom, by the way, used it illegally.

---

[55] Thomas Jefferson to George Fleming, December 29, 1815, National Archive: Founders Online, accessed October 28, 2021, https://founders.archives.gov/documents/Jefferson/03-09-02-0193.

[56] Clarke and Merlin, *Cannabis Evolution*, 449.

CHAPTER 7

Prohibition

I asked Tony Silvaggio how we went from presidents growing hemp to prospective presidents breaking the law by smoking it.

He responded, "Three important sources present a comprehensive social history of cannabis prohibition: Martin Booth's *Cannabis: A History*; Martin Lee's *Smoke Signals: A Social History of Marijuana*; and Nick Johnson's recent *Grass Roots: A History of Cannabis in the American West*.

"Many cannabis historians talk about the duality of the plant—it's fiber and flower; sacrament and scapegoat; helpful when a patient needs medicine, dangerous when a Mexican laborer needs to get through a long day of exploitation.

"Let's start in the 1700s and 1800s, when cannabis was a standard part of the American pharmacopeia, recommended by doctors for migraines, sore muscles, stomach cramps, alcoholism, post-natal depression, pain relief, diarrhea, and on and on. You could get it in any pharmacy. By the 1850s literally every pharmaceutical company in Britain and the US manufactured cannabis. You had it in tinctures, pills, cigarettes. You had Civil War vets using it to break their morphine addictions.

"Cannabis was discussed in medical journals. There were dozens of studies on the effectiveness of cannabis for pain relief. Even *The Lancet* had an article on medicinal uses of cannabis."

I told Tony about an 1843 article in *The Western Journal of Medicine and Surgery* that read, "The resin of the cannabis Indica is in general use as an intoxicating agent from the furthermost confines of India to Algiers. If this resin be swallowed, almost invariably the inebriation is of the most cheerful kind, causing the person to sing and dance, to eat food with great relish, and to seek aphrodisiac enjoyment. The intoxication lasts about three hours, when sleep supervenes; it is not followed by nausea or sickness, nor by any symptoms, except slight giddiness, worth recording."[1]

Tony laughed, then said, "In the US it wasn't for the most part used recreationally, although there were no laws against it."

He stopped a moment, then continued, "There were, however, at least a couple of medical challenges to cannabis becoming the physicians' drug of choice. The first is the difficulty of regulating dosage."

I thought of the times the juice had been too strong, and said, "Oh, yeah."

He said, "The other is that cannabis isn't injectable, which leads to the third problem, that it takes longer for cannabis to kick in than it does morphine, which can be more or less immediate. All of which led to physicians perceiving opiates and their synthetics—not cannabis—as the drugs of the future.

"Now," he said, "we need to bring in race and empire. In the nineteenth century the British started believing cannabis made workers lazy. So they criminalized it, first in the colonies: in India in 1838, Mauritius in 1840, Singapore in 1870, and so on."

"That's at the same time," I responded, "that the British were invading China to keep smuggling in opium."

"Criminalization had nothing to do with social benefit. The 1894 Indian Hemp Commission found that cannabis brought 'little harm' to society.

"Which doesn't alter the fact that in the late 1800s people around the world began to see drug use as a societal problem: remember, at that point cocaine, opium, and other drugs were legal in most countries, and I'm sure you've seen those old ads for heroin-laced children's cough syrups, or medicines like Mrs. Winslow's Soothing Syrup for

---

[1] Western Journal of Medicine and Surgery, 1843. Quoted in Matt Thompson, "The Mysterious History of 'Marijuana,'" NPR, July 22, 2013, accessed June 8, 2020, https://www.npr.org/sections/codeswitch/2013/07/14/201981025/the-mysterious-history-of-marijuana.

fussy babies. Sure, it put babies to sleep, but since the syrup contained alcohol mixed with 65 mg/ounce of morphine, sometimes the babies didn't wake up. And the stuff sold millions of bottles per year."

"Many of which were undoubtedly consumed by the mothers themselves."

"There are a couple of laws we have to talk about in order to understand how cannabis prohibition emerged. First, the Pure Food and Drug Act of 1906 required the listing of all ingredients in medicines. Prior to that, people hustled all sorts of tonics and drug cocktails. Then, the Harrison Narcotics Act of 1914 set a precedent as the first attempt by the feds to not merely list ingredients but regulate and tax pharmaceuticals. Non-medical consumption of narcotics was banned, and medical use was taxed.

"The point is that regulation of drugs wasn't necessarily motivated by economics or racism. There were health concerns. But there were a couple of problems. The first is that cannabis got lumped in with harder drugs, and the second is that prohibition was at the least informed by racism."

"How so?"

"It has to do with that dualism with which we perceive the plant—sacred and scapegoat, useful and dangerous—and how those groups in power tend to scapegoat and project menace onto those not in power."

"Like the Bible making Eve the scapegoat for getting humans kicked out of the Garden of Eden, or the standard patriarchal trope of women being dangerous temptresses?"

"Exactly. And this goes way back with weed as well. You and I both know that some Taoist sects used cannabis sacramentally, but other sects demonized weed and indigenous traditions as shamanic, which they said was a bad thing. Then later, Confucianism pretty much eliminated weed's sacramental use in China and then Japan. The Confucians believed that cannabis. . ." He got up, went to get a book, searched for a minute, then read, "'may cause rapid movements and under certain situations stimulate uncontrollable violence and criminal inclinations.'"

I responded, "But they didn't seem to be against opium and wine."

"Central to Confucianism is adherence to social norms, and it could be that someone sedated with opium might be less likely to challenge these norms. That can't necessarily be said of someone using cannabis."

I thought of the Scythians "shouting for joy," and figured Tony was onto something.

Tony said, "We could talk about the demonization of Chinese immigrants in the nineteenth century by associating them with opium, but let's move to the turn of the twentieth century when Mexican peasants, fleeing poverty and increasing social unrest, migrated into the border states. Prior to that, cannabis use had primarily been medicinal. Recreational smoking exploded—"

"Caught fire, you could say."

He chose to ignore me. "And the nativist movement in the US used this increase in recreational cannabis to scapegoat Mexicans, as they'd used opium to scapegoat Chinese."

And, I thought, as the ancient Arabs had used hashish to scapegoat the Hashashiyan. And then I remembered something else. I said, "Fifteen years ago I got an email from someone yelling at me in all CAPS because in some essay I hadn't used the word CANNABIS but instead MARIJUANA, which, I was told, was HATE SPEECH against MEXICANS and THE SACRED HERB."

"The argument is that in the nineteenth century weed was most commonly called cannabis, and in the early twentieth century the term was shifted intentionally to marijuana—a term used in Mexico, and of uncertain etymological origin[2]—specifically because those who opposed cannabis wanted to associate the plant with "Mexican-ness," and rile up both antidrug and anti-immigrant crusaders."

That reminded me of something Eric Schlosser wrote back in the nineties, in an article in The Atlantic, "The political upheaval in Mexico that culminated in the Revolution of 1910 led to a wave of Mexican immigration to states throughout the American Southwest. The prejudices and fears that greeted these peasant immigrants also extended

---

[2] One theory is that users of marijuana in Mexico named it after Mary, mother of Jesus, in order to appease or hold off Spanish colonizers who were attempting to crush ingestive use of marijuana, and to crush those who ingested it.

to their traditional means of intoxication: smoking marijuana. Police officers in Texas claimed that marijuana incited violent crimes, aroused a 'lust for blood,' and gave its users 'superhuman strength.' Rumors spread that Mexicans were distributing this 'killer weed' to unsuspecting American schoolchildren. Sailors and West Indian immigrants brought the practice of smoking marijuana to port cities along the Gulf of Mexico. In New Orleans newspaper articles associated the drug with African-Americans, jazz musicians, prostitutes, and underworld whites. 'The Marijuana Menace,' as sketched by antidrug campaigners, was personified by inferior races and social deviants."[3]

"In 1914," Tony continued, "El Paso became the first city to ban cannabis. The goal wasn't to make cannabis illegal as such, but to make life difficult for immigrants, who, because they worked low wage jobs, were accused of stealing people's livelihoods. Other cities followed."

I thought of some of the other claims made about marijuana. In Colorado the editor of a city newspaper wrote, "I wish I could show you what a small marihuana cigaret can do to one of our degenerate Spanish-speaking residents. That's why our problem is so great; the greatest percentage of our population is composed of Spanish-speaking persons, most of who [sic] are low mentally, because of social and racial conditions." And there's this, from the Los Angeles Times, "Not long ago a man who had smoked a marihuana cigarette attacked and killed a policeman and badly wounded three others; six policemen were needed to disarm him and march him to the police station where he had to be put into a straitjacket. Such occurrences are frequent. People who smoke marihuana finally lose their mind and never recover it, but their brains dry up and they die, most of times suddenly." A few years later, a member of California's State Board of Pharmacy wrote about other nonwhite immigrants, "Within the last year we in California have been getting a large influx of Hindoos and they have in turn started quite a demand for cannabis indica. They are a very undesirable lot and the habit is growing in California very fast; the fear is now that

---

[3] Eric Schlosser, "Reefer Madness," The Atlantic, August 1994, accessed June 8, 2020, https://www.theatlantic.com/magazine/archive/1994/08/reefer-madness/303476/.

it is not being confined to the Hindoos alone but that they are initiating our whites into this habit."[4]

Tony said, "The interesting thing is that at the time the biggest grower of cannabis in the US was the Department of Agriculture. They grew it for medicine so they didn't have to rely on foreign supplies.

"At that point states regulated the medical profession, while the feds imposed taxes. So California outlawed nonmedical use in the 1900s, and Texas outlawed marijuana altogether in 1919. By the mid-twenties, twelve states—Utah, Colorado, Wyoming, California, New Mexico, Nevada, Oregon, Washington, Maine, Vermont, Massachusetts, and Rhode Island—had banned it, and by 1933 half the country had banned the recreational use of cannabis.

"In 1930, the US government created the Federal Bureau of Narcotics, with Harry Anslinger as its first czar. He was rabidly antidrug, specifically antimarijuana. And he had a problem: his agency was young and underfunded near the start of the Great Depression, which means the government had more important things to spend money on than policing pot. So Anslinger put together an antimarijuana propaganda machine, running false stories in newspapers linking marijuana to rape and murder, creating phony science, and making laughably inaccurate documentaries. We've all heard of *Reefer Madness*, right?

"His plan worked not only in terms of funding but also legislation: in 1937 the feds passed the Marijuana Tax Act, which imposed a hundred-dollar tax—that'd be $1,800 today—on every marijuana exchange. If you didn't pay it, you got a steep fine for tax violation. It was a creative way to prohibit both medical and nonmedical uses of marijuana. So doctors would just not prescribe it. And yes, prior to that time doctors were prescribing it.

"Anslinger served through six presidential administrations. When he wanted to be tough on crime, he said smoking pot made you violent. During the Red Scare he said it made you docile and a pacifist. He pushed whatever narrative worked at the time, never mind the facts."

---

[4] All quoted in Matt Thompson, "The Mysterious History of 'Marijuana,'" *NPR*, July 22, 2013, accessed June 8, 2020, https://www.npr.org/sections/codeswitch/2013/07/14/201981025/the-mysterious-history-of-marijuana.

Tony got up, spent a few minutes rounding up and searching some other books, read a few Anslinger quotes:

"You smoke a joint and you're likely to kill your brother."[5]

"Marijuana is the most violence-causing drug in the history of mankind."[6]

"No one knows, when he places a marijuana cigarette to his lips, whether he will become a joyous reveler in a musical heaven, a mad insensate, a calm philosopher, or a murderer."[7]

"Reefer makes darkies think they're as good as white men."[8]

"There are 100,000 total marijuana smokers in the US, and most are Negroes, Hispanics, Filipinos and entertainers. Their Satanic music, jazz and swing, result from marijuana usage. This marijuana causes white women to seek sexual relations with Negroes, entertainers and any others."[9]

"If the hideous monster Frankenstein came face to face with marijuana, he would drop dead of fright."[10]

Tony said, "One of his most famous articles, called, 'Cannabis, the Assassin of Youth,' associated cannabis use with murder and depravity.

"People were scared of him, like they were scared of J. Edgar Hoover. He was a proponent of the sword: punitive measures to control what he thought was deviant behavior.

"He did, however have his challengers. In the 1940s, New York mayor Fiorello LaGuardia commissioned a report on how cannabis affected the city. The report debunked all Anslinger's claims. It found no link between cannabis and crime, juvenile delinquency, or violence and also noted the medical benefits of cannabis. This incensed Anslinger, who used his influence to get the American Medical

---

[5] Elizabeth Brown and George Barganier, *Race and Crime: Geographies of Injustice* (Oakland: University of California Press, 2018), 212.

[6] Jack Herer, Jeanie Cabarga, and Jeanie Herer, *The Emperor Wears No Clothes: Hemp and the Marijuana Conspiracy* (Austin: Ah Ha Publishing, 1985), 59.

[7] Harry Anslinger, "Marijuana: The Assassin of Youth," *The American Magazine,* July 1937, 18.

[8] Brown and Barganier, *Race and Crime,* 212.

[9] Herer, Cabarga, and Herer, *The Emperor Wears No Clothes,* 29.

[10] Martin Booth, *Cannabis: A History* (New York: Picador, 2003), 177–178.

Association and the Pharmaceutical Trade Association to publicly criticize the report and get it buried.

"In the 1950s he accelerated his assault on cannabis, advocating for and getting passed the Boggs Act, which laid out minimum sentencing guidelines for cannabis possession: first offense, two to five years; second offense, five to ten years; third offense, ten to twenty years. For a joint! In 1956 they revised the Boggs Act and called it the 1956 Narcotics Control Act. This increased maximum prison times to ten years for your first offense, twenty for your second, and thirty for your third.

"Even if most got the minimum, the possibility of doing the maximum scared a lot of people out of it."

"To this we have to add the stigma."

"And so far, we've only been talking about the feds. Over the decades various states passed prohibition laws, with those in the South being the most strict. In some states simple possession could get you ninety-nine years. In Georgia a second offense could get you the death penalty. I've never heard that anyone got death for simple possession, but it was on the books."

"At that point, what percent of people in the US were smoking pot?"

"Certainly nothing like today. Among some groups—Mexican laborers, jazz musicians and fans, beatniks, a few other populations—there was a fair amount of usage, but in the fifties it wasn't for the most part in the vocabulary of the general populace."

"Was the available marijuana grown domestically or imported?"

"The majority came from Mexico. But of course, some people saved seeds to grow. And some immigrants brought seeds with them and grew them for personal use. For example, Syrian refugees in the 1800s brought seeds and planted them in their yards."

"Just like someone might do with pomegranates or grapes."

"Exactly," he said.

Tony said, "In 1961 you had the United Nations Convention on Narcotic Drugs, an international agreement prohibiting recreational cannabis worldwide."

"So if, say, Argentina wanted to legalize cannabis, it was prohibited from doing so?"

"Think about the International Monetary Fund and World Bank Structural Adjustment Programs. Same stuff. In order to get aid, countries needed to engage in cannabis eradication programs.

"The UN Convention on Narcotic Drugs created an enforcement arm called the International Narcotics Control Board. So you have international efforts to police narcotics and specifically cannabis.[11]

"Now we're into the late sixties. In 1969 Nixon ramped up the War on Drugs, again specifically making the link between crime, drugs, and black and brown people. Bruce Barcott, in his book *Weed the People*, documented the absurdities Nixon believed about cannabis, for example that communists were pushing it because it encouraged homosexuality, immorality, and crime.

"In 1970, the US passed the Controlled Substances Act, which was the national implementation of the UN Convention on Narcotic Drugs. Among other things, this put in place the scheduling or categorization of drugs, where Schedule I is the most restricted, through Schedule V. Schedule I drugs are declared to have no medical use, a high potential for abuse, and extreme safety concerns. Heroin is a Schedule I drug. So, they said, is cannabis. For comparison: cocaine, meth, fentanyl, PCP, and Nembutal—mainly used these days for assisted suicide and for putting down your beloved pets—are all Schedule II. Alcohol and tobacco are explicitly excluded from the law's definition of a drug.

"There were, thank goodness, some challenges to that scheduling. The Shafer Commission debunked it, found there was little health risk from cannabis, and that that there was no evidence to substantiate the theory that cannabis is a gateway to harder drugs. The Shafer Commission recommended cannabis be taken completely off the list of scheduled drugs, and that it be decriminalized. But Nixon buried that. The findings were never enforced.

---

[11] Speaking of international law enforcement and cannabis, after the Six Day War, Mossad had a plan code-named Operation Blade to buy Lebanese hash and sell it to Egyptian soldiers, with the hope they'd be too stoned to fight.

"The Controlled Substances Act was part of the larger Comprehensive Drug Abuse Prevention and Control Act, which also removed the mandatory minimum sentences and penalties for pot. This was frankly because a lot of white college kids were getting busted and sentenced to real time, which wasn't sitting well with Nixon's constituency.

"In 1973, Nixon created the Drug Enforcement Agency. Because at the time the majority of cannabis consumed in the US was low quality weed from Mexico, Nixon spent hundreds of millions of dollars on interdiction efforts, including stationing agents at the border and spraying paraquat on crops. We talked before about how this led to an increase in both imports from other countries and domestic production.

"Let's move to the eighties with Reagan's militarization of cannabis eradication and his even more punitive approach than his predecessors. He signed the Comprehensive Crime Control Act of 1984, which allowed the assets forfeitures we talked about earlier, which in turn helped finance military-style policing of cities. He also used federal forces to spray paraquat in US National Forests. In many ways the Reagan years were the low point for marijuana's legal status in the United States, at least at the federal level."

I thought about cannabis prohibitions, and how these prohibitions ultimately fail. I thought of something Dr. Louis Lewin, founder of ethnobotany, wrote in his phenomenal 1924 *Phantastica: A Classic Survey on the Use and Abuse of Mind-Altering Plants*: "It is recorded that in the year 1378 the Emir Soudoun Sheikhouni tried to end the abuse of Indian hemp consumption among the poorer classes by having all plants of this description in Joneima destroyed and imprisoning all the hemp-eaters. He ordered, moreover, that all those who were convicted of eating the plant should have their teeth pulled out, and many were subjected to this punishment. But by 1393 the use of this substance in Arabian territory had increased."[12]

Both the plant and those who love it are nothing if not tenacious.

---

[12] Louis Lewin, M.D., *Phantastica: A Classic Survey on the Use and Abuse of Mind-Altering Plants* (New York: E. P. Dutton, 1964), 107.

Legalization:
Prohibition 2.0

Tony said,[1] "In August, 1964, twenty-eight-year-old Lowell Eggemeier walked into the San Francisco Hall of Justice, lit a joint, and said to police, 'I am starting a campaign to legalize marijuana smoking. I wish to be arrested.' He teamed up with an ultraconservative libertarian attorney to argue the constitutionality of cannabis prohibition. He lost the case, spent a year in prison, and had a felony on his record but was responsible for starting the movement to reform cannabis laws.

"Eggemeier wasn't a hippy. He had short hair and a neat beard. He just believed the government didn't have the right to tell him what to do with his body. After his release from prison he withdrew from politics, including legalization activism, and returned to hanging out with his beloved dogs.

"His case helped bring about a group called LeMar, for Legalize Marijuana—"

I said, "I wonder if they were stoned when they came up with that clever name."

Tony responded, "At least they didn't call it MarijLega." Then he said, "They had several chapters across the US. These weren't your typical professional, well-funded, social-change organizations but honest-to-goodness volunteer, grassroots groups. They produced position papers on cannabis law and gave people data on arrests.

---

[1] Tony would like to note that a lot of the info in this chapter comes from a book by Emily Dufton called *Grass Roots: The Rise and Fall and Rise of Marijuana in America* (New York: Basic Books/Hachette Book Group, 2017).

"Then in 1969 another group emerged, also on the West Coast, called Amorphia, founded by hemp advocates who sold hemp rolling papers to fund the legalization movement. In 1972 they backed Prop 19, the California Marijuana Initiative, that would have allowed cultivation and personal use. It failed, getting 33 percent of the vote, which wasn't too bad considering that between 1968 and 1972 polls consistently showed support for marijuana legalization in the United States at about 15 percent. Prop 19 was instrumental because it was the first cannabis-law reform initiative in the world.

"One reason I keep emphasizing that to this point marijuana legalization efforts were truly grassroots is that the transformation of the legalization movement presages the more recent transformation we've discussed with growing and distributing, that is, from mom and pop culture to corporate cannabis culture, in that the first organizations that developed to challenge cannabis prohibition laws were grassroots, and they were consumed over the next decades by those that were more professionalized and mainstream.

"In this case you also had a geographical split: West-Coast and East-Coast organizations. In the West you had LeMar and Amorphia. Their approach was full-on legalization. In 1970 in the East an attorney named Keith Stroup formed a group called NORML: the National Organization to Reform Marijuana Laws. The group's early money came from Hugh Hefner and *Playboy*, which eventually provided hundreds of thousands of dollars for this organization. NORML took a different approach, arguing for reduced sentencing and decriminalization instead of outright legalization.

"Part of this difference had to do with culture and geography. Groups like NORML took the traditional lobbying approach and relied heavily on thinktanks. They looked at polling data. They queried members of congress to gauge support for initiatives."

I said, "At this point, even though it was illegal, marijuana was pretty popular, right? Paul McCartney wrote "Got to Get You Into My Life" about pot. Jimi Hendrix toked up onstage. And by 1978, when I started going to concerts, people routinely passed joints down the rows."

He responded, "In the 1950s, the average American didn't even know what marijuana was. Then the sixties and seventies—during and after the Vietnam War and the counter-culture revolution in the US— were a time of interesting contradictions. On one hand, marijuana was everywhere. You heard about it in music. You saw it in films like *Easy Rider* or the Cheech and Chong movies. But at the same time, you had *Hawaii Five-O*, *Adam 12*, *Dragnet*—TV shows where mad, mad reefer madness was happening.

"By 1972, LeMar, Amorphia, and NORML had merged. NORML became the primary group fighting for legislative change at the local, state, and federal levels."

Tony said, "You can't talk about marijuana legalization efforts without talking about the 1971 book, *Marihuana Reconsidered*, by Harvard Medical School professor Dr. Lester Grinspoon."[2]

"I grow Dr. Grinspoon!"

"A legendary strain. What's it like?"

"It's pure sativa—"

"So it takes forever to mature—"

"A hundred days." I said, "The buds smell like rancid fat, unfortunately. But the effect is interesting. It's not like Trainwreck, which is basically a sledge hammer to the front of your brain. If you smoke Grinspoon, then distract yourself, you don't notice anything. You think, 'What is this crap?' But if after you smoke it, you, say, sit still by a forested stream, it makes subtle yet profound changes in your perception. Depth becomes tangible, as though you can hold distance itself in your hand, and even in a tangle you see each branch clearly. You hear and recognize birdsongs and the calls of insects you never before noticed and can almost discern the melody and harmonies in the sounds of the stream."

"Grinspoon himself underwent profound changes in his perception," Tony said. "Concerned about increases in cannabis usage in the

---

[2] Lester Grinspoon, M.D., *Marihuana Reconsidered* (Cambridge, MA: Harvard University Press, 1971).

sixties, he set out to thoroughly review and publicize medical evidence on the dangers of marijuana. But he found there was little empirical evidence to back the claims of prohibition drug warriors. His book made clear not only that the government was feeding us hogwash, but demonstrated how they were doing it.

"He wrote a number of books advocating for medical use of cannabis and referred to what was taking place with cannabis research as psychopharmacological McCarthyism. His work broke open the conversation about medical uses of pot."

Tony continued, "In 1972, Holland had its own version of the Shafer Commission, called the Bond Commission, which had similar findings that cannabis isn't harmful and should be decriminalized. Unlike the US, the Dutch implemented the recommendations, and while, technically, cannabis remained illegal, the laws weren't enforced. That led to the pot and coffee shops we've all heard about, and some of us have visited.

"Back to the US. In 1975, there was the famous case of *Robert Randall v. U.S.* Randall was an English professor in DC who'd been told in his early twenties he'd be blind by thirty because of glaucoma. He found that cannabis significantly helped his condition, so he grew some plants in his back yard. He got arrested, then sued the feds—everyone from the FDA to the DEA; to the DOJ; to the National Institute on Drug Abuse to the Department of Health, Education, and Welfare—and won using the common-law doctrine of necessity, in this case medical necessity. The feds created the Compassionate Investigational New Drug Program and grew marijuana at a farm at the University of Mississippi to supply him—and eventually a few other people—with pot. He became the first person since 1937 to have a prescription for marijuana."

"How much did they give him?"

"Three hundred joints per month, if you can believe it. Admittedly, they made him sue and sue and sue, and they made him fill out a bazillion arcane forms, and the pot was brown and seedy schwag, but still. . .

"In 1976, he and his partner founded a grassroots volunteer group called the Alliance for Cannabis Therapeutics to push for medical cannabis in the US."

*

"All of this—and cannabis culture in general—was preparing society for legalization and showing that society was in many ways ready for it. In 1974, Tom Forçade, using money made through illegal pot sales, published *High Times*. It was supposed to be a one-off spoof of *Playboy*, substituting weed for women, including a centerfold of a plant, but it was so popular they turned it into a news/cheerleading magazine for cannabis culture. Within a couple of years, it had a circulation of a half-million, rivalling *Rolling Stone* and *National Lampoon*."

I said, "I was interviewed once for *High Times*, about fed surveillance capabilities. To thank me for the interview, they gave me a T-shirt that reads, 'All My Heroes Have FBI Files.'

"Of course, this was back when FBI files meant something, before the surveillance state made it so everybody has one."

Tony said, "The Oregon state legislature decriminalized personal amounts of marijuana in 1973. A bunch of states followed: Colorado, Ohio, Alaska, California, Maine, Minnesota, South Dakota, Mississippi, New York, North Carolina, Nebraska. In all those states personal possession became basically a civil fine, like a parking ticket.

"In 1976, Jimmy Carter was elected president. He embraced decriminalization, tried to implement the Shafer report recommendations, and had the feds back off on prosecutions.

"One of Carter's drug policy advisors was Dr. Peter Bourne. He supported decriminalization. He became friends with some cannabis reform activists, including Keith Stroup, founder/director of NORML. One Christmas, Bourne was at a NORML party, doing lines of coke. Reporters heard about this and wanted to know more. Stroup tried to pressure Bourne into pressuring Carter into stopping the spraying of paraquat. He got rebuffed—either by Bourne or Carter, I don't know—got pissed about it, then outed Bourne to the press. Terrible, terrible move. He got Bourne fired, set back the decrim movement and, in fact, got kicked out of his own organization for being a snitch.

"In the late seventies Dennis Peron pushed for Prop W in San Francisco that would have prohibited the police and the district attorney from arresting or prosecuting people for cultivating, possessing, or using marijuana. The proposition passed and would have become law in San Francisco, but George Moscone, the famous liberal mayor, and the equally famous and equally liberal city council member Harvey Milk, were both murdered.[3]

"The new mayor was Dianne Feinstein—now a longtime senator from California—and she refused to enact the proposition.

"By this point marijuana and its accessories were everywhere. You could buy papers, bongs, gas masks attached to bongs, and other drug paraphernalia at corner stores, record stores, bodegas, head shops.

"All of this cannabis normalization led to a powerful prohibitionist countermovement that started in Atlanta, Georgia, in 1976, then quickly went nationwide. It was a true grassroots movement of parents scared shitless about the rise of drug culture, and what it could do to their children. The first few parents educated and organized more parents, who educated and organized more parents, who put together manuals and conferences on how to stop the scourge of drugs. By the eighties there were 4,000 of these groups across the country. They were able to stop and even roll back some of the decrim efforts."

"You could argue they're one reason—among many—Reagan was elected."

"You could also argue they succeeded, at least for a while: as a result of their work adolescent drug use reached an all-time low.

"And of course, by the eighties the organizations of parents were no longer run by parents but had been taken over by non-profit professionals.

"It doesn't matter whether we're talking about the environmental movement, the organic farming movement, the marijuana farming movement, the marijuana legalization movement, the movement of parents against adolescent drug use—it's the same story. 'Industrial complex,' as in 'military-industrial complex,' is an overused term, but it fits: the non-profit-industrial complex. The cannabis-industrial complex.

---

[3] By a former police officer.

"By the eighties this movement was funded by the feds, and by pharmaceutical, alcohol, and tobacco companies to the tune of hundreds of millions of dollars, with organizations like the Partnership for a Drug-Free America, the Office of National Drug Control, National Families in Action, and the Drug Abuse Resistance Education program—"

"Which I always thought had a terrible acronym, not only because one kid could dare another to take drugs, but also because to this day I can never remember what the acronym stands for, and the only thing that comes to mind is Drugs Are Really Exciting. If even someone like me who never takes drugs thinks that's what it stands for—"

"It's a terrible acronym," Tony agreed, then said, "And as always, when money talks, government listens—even when a lot of the money comes from the government. That's why the eighties saw the proliferation of drug testing, such that any worker whose job was connected to the feds had to take a piss test. And any contractor that wanted to do business with the feds had to likewise police their employees.

"Let's move forward to 1991. San Francisco, in the midst of the AIDS epidemic, passed Prop P, which disallowed enforcement of laws against marijuana for medical purposes. Dennis Peron, who had pushed for Prop W, opened the San Francisco Buyers Club to provide medicine to those with AIDS or other serious medical conditions. A couple of years later the Women's Alliance for Medical Marijuana got a similar measure passed in Santa Cruz.

"As well as the SF Buyers Club, lots of underground dispensaries sprang up, where they'd tell their patients, 'Today we're at this location, so come and get your pot. Tomorrow we'll be at that location, and the day after at another.' But Peron wasn't going to go underground. He was determined to challenge the laws.

"This made him a target for state and federal governments, both of which repeatedly raided his club and other dispensaries. This was under Republican Governor Wilson and Democrat President Clinton. And because these dispensaries were prohibited by the feds from using banks, they had to deal in large amounts of cash, which made them vulnerable not only to government seizures but to common criminals.

"The urban myth—which may or may not have an element of truth—is that the state raids on dispensaries so incensed Peron and others that they vowed to change state law.[4] They knew the governor would veto anything passed by the legislature, so they decided to go directly to the people of California.

"They quickly got 700,000 signatures for Prop 215, the Compassionate Use Act, which then passed with 56 percent of the vote.

"The proposition was intentionally written to be open-ended: allowing marijuana for any medical condition for which marijuana provides relief, everything from AIDS to Crohn's, to migraines, to aches and pains, to whatever. All you had to do was get a doctor to issue you a certificate."

"What percent," I asked, "of the certificates do you think were for legitimate medical conditions, and what percent were excuses to get high? I've heard so many jokes about this, especially from growers who used the law as an excuse for commercial grows."

"That's a fair question. Early on, not many, since the feds threatened doctors with losing their licenses if caught prescribing pot to patients. But a handful of doctors got around that by writing not 'prescriptions' but 'recommendations.' A patient could go in, pay a doctor a hundred dollars, and get the 'recommendation.' And sure, some people used it for cancer, but Peron later stated that Prop 215 effectively legalized cannabis in that it gave people an affirmative defense for growing, possessing, and smoking pot. He was exaggerating, since people were still thrown in jail for it. But it was a major step. It also allowed 'caregivers' to grow plants for consumption by others and didn't set a limit on the number of plants. That created a problem for regulators and law

---

[4] I spoke with one medical marijuana advocate who said, "When I explain Peron and Prop 215 to people, I always highlight that Dennis was a humanitarian and Prop 215 reflects that good nature. I think 215 is about sixty pages long. It is easy to read and understand. I contrast this with the current law providing for legalization—Prop 64—which was written by corporate lawyers, and which I believe is about six hundred pages long. For me at least, it requires a lawyer hired at $420/hr. to translate/understand it. I am not at all a policy person or a writer, but it seems as though most of our laws have gone from being somewhat understandable to being written in an elite language that requires a $200,000+ degree to even remotely understand."

enforcement, because how many plants does a person need for medicine? One? Two? A hundred?"

"I'm a good example of this confusion, since my primary method of consumption is juiced leaves, and it takes a tremendous number of plants to make not very much juice."

"And people used that confusion to grow thousands of plants."

I asked, "Wasn't this then in some ways the golden age of the cottage industry? Because it was easier under the law to rationalize having a hundred plants than having entire city blocks of greenhouses in Santa Barbara. You still had those legal barriers to economies of scale."

"The barriers were not only legal but also cultural. Santa Barbara didn't have a pre-existing cannabis-growing culture. The Emerald Triangle did. And now people could grow indoors without much stealth—get yourself a card from a doctor and grow in your spare room. Here in Humboldt you'd have neighborhoods where 70 percent of the homes contained grows.

"Another change was that people could now talk more openly about weed. It became not uncommon to overhear people at restaurants or grocery stores talking about their grows. And people started flashing cash. There was less fear The Man was coming to get you, because you had a legal out.

"People took advantage of every loophole they could, for example, buying and selling medical cards. More than a few big growers photocopied these cards and sold or rented them to customers.

"The vagueness of the proposition also created the perfect conditions for environmental abuses, in part because its vagueness made it difficult to put in place licensing or regulatory systems. There were no rules regarding where or how you could grow, what you could put in the soil, how much water you could use. Large-scale indoor and outdoor cannabis grows took over the Emerald Triangle.

"The beauty of 215 was that it gave people freedom from police suppression and helped the cannabis community to come out more in the open. But it also brought in a lot of bad actors, people who took advantage of a system that wasn't necessarily meant to facilitate people becoming multimillionaires.

"In 2003, California Senate Bill 420—and yes, that was its real number—was written to at least somewhat deal with Prop 215's ambiguities regarding growing and distributing cannabis by giving counties the legal right to set their own rules. Predictably, counties in the Emerald Triangle opted for the most liberal rules allowed by the state. For example, they allowed cannabis cultivators to grow up to ninety-nine plants per card."

After Senate Bill 420, the county where I live, Del Norte, set the limit for how many plants an individual can grow for medicinal purposes at ninety-nine.

There are those who, believe it or not, found that number excessive.

So the county Board of Supervisors wanted to reduce that number to six. Before the board could do that, however, it needed to hold a public hearing.

The hearing was a lesson in participatory democracy. The meeting room was packed with angry growers and users, clamoring against the possibility of the Board of Supervisors taking away their medicine (or, in some cases, their pot). Had the members of the board voted that night to lower the number of plants a person can grow, they would have had a hard time escaping the room.

That was participatory democracy in action, in all its glorious messiness.

All that said, the evening broke my heart, because the room was packed to protect people's access to marijuana, but when it comes to things like protecting salmon, maybe four or five people will show up.

I am unutterably saddened that people love marijuana more than they love salmon, more than they love any part of the wild world.

I shared this with a small cannabis grower who responded, "It's not that people love cannabis more than salmon. I think it's true they love money more than salmon. They are defending their means of making money, earning a living, which within this system means surviving.

"I'll tell you my experience of board of supervisors meetings. Where I live, the board of supervisors' meetings were a sad joke. The rooms

were full of people trying to save their livelihoods and the local economy: the public comment meetings weren't about the plant so much
as about economic survival. I found there was always a chilling discon-
nect with these boards; a large part of the population of these towns,
some with practically zero industry, kept their towns economically
lubricated with cannabis dollars. From my perspective as one of those
smaller cannabis business owners, I was routinely enraged at the disre-
gard and disrespect our board of supervisors showed us. We brought
so much money into our towns. When the law was changing in this
county, I spent hours in these board of supervisors' meetings listening
to well-written and intelligent statements from local farmers—farmers
who were rightly terrified to show their faces in public in connection
with cannabis—pleading and providing guidance for fair regulation.
And consistently, these statements weren't taken seriously. The supervisors didn't need to listen because they'd already made backdoor deals
with a few farmers and corporations. The farmers who were not in the
select few at the back door got the bitter taste of how public comment
at the meetings makes no difference to the outcome of policy when
enrichment is at stake.

"That said, I don't disagree with your basic point. These days, to
acquire a license now in the community where I live, a cannabis business must present in front of a committee how they'll bring in tax
dollars. Wouldn't it be great if all businesses had to present to the board
how they'll do good for the natural world? This is another example of
how the exchange of dollars has undermined relationship.

"And of course, I'm with you regarding the devastating lack of out-
rage and support when salmon need protection.

"But as we know, money talks, and we can basically just replace the
word *cannabis* with the word *dollar* and we would all know how the
legal structures will end up looking.

"I guess my bottom line is that capitalism is psychotic, and I wish
I could snap my fingers and heal the collective human psyche that
is addicted to this system. There will be a day when the majority of
humans will do whatever it takes to save the natural world. What it
will take to get to that point will probably involve a *lot* of suffering.

Humans have damaged the natural world so much that it's not possible to rely on the local wild landscape for survival. When we're forced to make that jump, I believe cannabis will be an essential plant."

Tony said, "Allowing cannabis cultivators to grow up to ninety-nine plants per Prop 215 card, and to 'caregive' as many patients as they wanted, created a kind of Wild West for cannabis cultivators. Not only did it increase the size of both indoor and outdoor grows, but it also allowed the employment of new agricultural practices like growing outdoor year-round with supplemental electric lights powered by diesel generators.

"The industry—even the cottage industry—was requiring more energy inputs, more water, more fertilizers, more conversion of forests to cannabis farms.

"Every year from 2000 until eventual legalization saw an increase in marijuana production in this region, which means increases in harm to watersheds from the cumulative impact of thousands of growers, including massive industrial cannabis farms."

I asked, "What do these farms do to salmon? I've known multiple growers who pull water directly from salmon-bearing streams."

Tony responded, "California Fish and Game estimates that because of the tens of thousands of grows—yes, tens of thousands—cannabis cultivation can take as much as about 50 percent of flow during the driest part of the summer and completely dewater some streams, including those previously home to endangered steelhead and salmon populations.

"As much as I'd like to put all the blame on huge greenhouses and even more huge outdoor grows, fifty or a hundred small grows in one watershed can just as effectively harm the streams. Right now, I could drive you over to see scores of small farms pumping water directly out of streams. Salmon need that water.

"And remember, these are lands and streams already hammered by decades of logging."

I shared *this* exchange with another cannabis grower. She responded, "All monocrop farming is terrible. So I'm happy to criticize cannabis.

It's true that cannabis uses a lot of water to farm. But grapes use more water, and I believe if we are to discuss the farming of mind-altering substances, I think we should move from solely criticizing cannabis to including grape farming for wine.

"Many of the grape growers in Mendocino pump water from the creeks, and Fish and Game looks the other way, but a cannabis farmer who gets caught pumping water from the creek gets locked up. I think any pumping of water from creeks is terrible, but I do like to point out the preferential treatment received by grape growers, many of whom are part of the regional good-ol'-boys network. I used to grow cannabis on a vineyard and overheard conversations the owner had with his son about how untouchable they are because the winegrowers are in with the politicians. I knew some vineyard owners who, when discovered, blamed their own illegal grows on their Mexican vineyard workers.

"I think one of the most dangerous creatures on the planet is a drunk male human. Why aren't we regulating vineyards like we do cannabis? Why don't boards of supervisors limit how many grape plants a person can own?"

Tony said, "I started investigating the environmental effects of cannabis cultivation in 2010. Pretty much everybody I spoke with who grew weed didn't want to talk about it. They knew it was going on, but *they* didn't do it. Everybody else did. Those in the cannabis policy reform movement were even worse—cheerleaders who could admit no possible wrong in their community: 'Cannabis is all organic and our cannabis community always does the right thing.' The best interpretation you could put on this is that they were clueless. When testing began in 2012 and 2013, the weed was coming back dirty. There were pesticides all over the place.

"When I started this research, I'd ask cops, game wardens, and so on: 'When you busted this grow in the forest, what chemicals were there? How many pounds? Did you take photos of the pesticides, herbicides, and fertilizers?' And they never had any idea. They didn't care. All they cared about was how many plants they pulled up, because plant count was all that mattered toward that sweet, sweet government money for next year's budget. So they regularly left the chemicals there, and certainly didn't rehabilitate the land.

"They didn't even start collecting data on pesticide and fertilizer use in trespass grows on National Forest land until 2014. The government doesn't care, which is why it makes me sick these days to hear cops talking about how they need to be in the forest protecting it from marijuana growers. They never cared before. They certainly didn't care when MAXXAM/Pacific Lumber was cutting the hell out of old growth redwood forests, and cops were beating the shit out of those of us trying to stop it. Hell, they still don't care about Green Diamond Resource Company clearcutting and spraying pesticides. They didn't—and don't—care about the wine industry taking water and destroying the land. But when it comes to marijuana grows, we're supposed to believe they care."

I asked, "Can you talk about the effects of pesticides on Humboldt marten?"

"There are a number of pesticides—many smuggled in because they're illegal in the US—widely used by cultivators doing trespass grows on wild public lands.

"Some of these grows are immense. A hundred thousand plants. Most are smaller. They'll lay a kill zone of insecticides and rodenticide around the entire grow, so much poison that anything crossing the line dies.

"In 2013, ecologists found Carbofuran at over 70 percent of marijuana grow sites on public lands in California.[5] It's a horrible chemical. A single grain will kill a bird, millions of whom have been killed by it. It's used illegally in Kenya to kill lions; they pour it on a carcass, the lion eats it, and dies. It's considered a significant threat to entire populations. Carbofuran bioaccumulates, killing those who eat those it has killed. It can kill on contact, not only by ingestion. And to humans it's one of the three most toxic agricultural chemicals in use anywhere.

---

5   "Toxic Pesticide Use Rising At Illegal California Pot Farms," Associated Press, *KPIX CBS SF Bay Area*, May 29, 2018, accessed December 1, 2020, https://sanfrancisco.cbslocal.com/2018/05/29/toxic-pesticide-carbofuran-illegal-pot-farms/.

"It's not the only chemical used. There's also a lot of anticoagulant rodenticide use. It's rat poison that has flavor enhancers mixed in to cause animals to eat it. Imagine you're walking down the street and smell a barbecue. What do you do? You think of food and you walk toward it.

"You have all these idiots in public forests, dropping in thousands of plants, then putting out poisons that attract wild animals from all over the forest."

"Bears, for example," I said, "can smell food literally for miles."

"All these animals eat the stuff and get killed from the inside. They bleed out. It's a slow death, during which they become disoriented. And what happens to animals stumbling around the forest? They get eaten by other animals who then bleed out, stumble around the forest, and get eaten by yet other animals. Rinse and repeat. It's devastating.

"And this shit stays active in the soil for well over a year.

"Mourad Gabriel was one of the first researchers to uncover this in the Sierra Nevada. He noticed a high rate of deaths among fishers miles and miles away from any humans and eventually figured out they were eating poisoned rodents. And it's not just fishers, but basically anyone who eats, including critically endangered Humboldt martens, of whom only 300 individuals remain in three distinct and separated populations of a hundred each. And illegal marijuana farming is, along with other habitat loss, road mortality, and trapping, one of the four primary causes of mortality."

"The other environmental harm I want to ask about is deforestation for marijuana grows."

"Which is interesting in itself. Back when pot was illegal a lot of pot was shade-grown, in part because people were afraid of being spotted from helicopters. It's a skill to grow weed that way.

"These days you can see clearcuts in Google Earth. You scroll a little and see a clearcut. It's marijuana. You scroll a little more, and it's a clearcut by a timber company. My point is not to excuse the cannabis clearcuts, but to make clear the cumulative impacts of extractive industry after extractive industry."

"I don't think," I said, "the forest cares whether the clearcut is done by MAXXAM, Green Diamond, or the groovy marijuana farmer; nor do salmon care whether their stream is dewatered by those growing wine or pot."

"All of this is why in 2015 California passed bills to regulate medical cannabis, giving oversight to three government agencies. The Department of Food and Agriculture regulated cultivation, the Department of Public Health dealt with manufacturing, and the Consumer Affairs Department was in charge of testing and distribution of cannabis. The laws passed in 2015 provided, for the first time since the implementation of Prop 215, an outline of environmental protections for cannabis cultivation, detailing guidelines on water protection, pesticides, other environmental problems we've come to associate with cannabis cultivation, and product testing. Honestly, I think it helped small growers. For example, restricting the use of pesticides effectively banned large-scale commercial medical cannabis.[6]

"In the meantime, you had states like Colorado and Washington passing full legalization.

"This brings us to 2016 and Proposition 64, the Adult Use of Marijuana Act, legalizing cannabis in California. In its run-up it was heralded by environmental activists and policy-makers as the gold standard of cannabis legislation because it funded conservation, restoration, and the enforcement of environmental laws. And it was unprecedented to see an initiative have regulatory mandates specifying permits for every type of cannabis commerce, as well as heavy fines for noncompliance. These regulations and fines would later become a real problem, particularly for small growers.

"A lot of small growers had concerns about legalization, mostly having to do with the understanding that when you remove barriers to economies of scale, there's no way a cottage industry can compete with the big moneyed interests.

"One way the bill's promoters tried to counter that was by telling us the bill would give small growers a five-year head start in the regulated market by forbidding licenses for cannabis farms larger than one acre

---

[6] I shared this with a cannabis activist who told me, "A lot of them still use systemic pesticides and get away with it, even with today's 'rigorous' testing."

for five years. This would allow small farmers time to learn how to jump through regulatory hoops before big corporate growers jumped in.

"In 2016, there were a lot of marijuana legalization initiatives competing to be put on the ballot in California, and Prop 64 ended up at the top in great measure because it was promoted and funded by a lot of rich organizations and individuals, like then-Lieutenant Governor (now Governor) Gavin Newsom, and the former president of Facebook, Sean Parker. They brought their dog and pony show to the Emerald Triangle, toured small farms, and told us they'd protect the cottage industry here.

"The law we passed contained the five-year head start provision, and also an outright ban on large operations.

"Given the big money involved, none of us should be surprised we got a bait-and-switch. After passage, as they drafted final regulations, what I call Cannacrats joined with neoliberal Democratic politicians to do what the system does and aligned themselves with Big Canna (large private cannabis interests), young techbros, and all the other big money speculators who have no relationship to the plant, no traditional cannabis culture, and really no care for anything other than the number of digits they see on their checks.

"Before the proposition went into effect, they removed the five-year ban on big farms, inserting a loophole that removed protection for small farmers and removed limits on large farms altogether. In the drafting of the regs, there had been big arguments over whether the largest allowable farms should be one acre, ten acres, or somewhere in between. Then when the regs were published—what do you know—there was no limit whatsoever."

"American democracy in action."

"It happens every time, in every field, doesn't it?"

"And even on the smallest scale," I said. "Decades ago, I was asked to be part of a gathering of policy-makers and lobbyists to discuss children's health issues. The organizers specifically asked me to advocate for the environment—children of all species, I suppose. The thing was a nightmare. Before the end of the weekend the children's health advocates were literally yelling at me that I was wasting their time talking about environmental destruction and that environmentalists have it much easier than children's health advocates, to which I should have responded—and would have had I not by then grown disgusted with the whole process—by asking them when was the last time someone framed an issue not as 'owls versus jobs' but 'babies versus jobs.' Worse than this, though, was the sleaziness of a lobbyist who ran some of the breakout sessions. He smiled to my face while he wrote down my concerns, and then every time we'd return to the main group I'd discover that before he left the small room, he'd erased everything I'd said."

"That was a nice introduction to the public input process, wasn't it?"

"It's the same as public comments on Forest Service timber sales, and pretty much everything else. The corporate anthropologist Jane Anne Morris wrote, 'Corporate persons have constitutional rights to due process and equal protection that human persons, affected citizens, don't have. For noncorporate human citizens there's a democracy theme park where we can pull levers on voting machines and talk into microphones at hearings. But don't worry, they're not connected to anything and nobody is listening 'cept for us. What regulatory law regulates is citizen input, not corporate behavior.'"[7]

Tony continued, "Suddenly you had 10,000 farmers in the Emerald Triangle having to compete with Big Canna backed by the Cannacrats and the full power of the state. You had all of these farmers doing their best to fit into the legal system, trying to get into the permitting structure, but they couldn't afford the fees or compete with the big farms.

"The California Growers Association—an association of small, organic, back-to-the-land farmers—sued the state. But during the process of waiting for all the legal pieces to move, the state just went ahead and started handing out licenses to big cannabis companies."

"It's the same every time, isn't it?"

---

[7] Jane Anne Morris, "Help! I've Been Colonized and I Can't Get Up (1998) (Take a lawyer and an expert to a hearing and call me in a decade . . .): Are Regulatory Agencies a Good Thing?" Democracy Theme Park, http://democracythemepark. org/help-ive-been-colonized-and-i-cant-get-up/.

"Every fucking time. Back in the timber wars, we'd go to court to get a restraining order, which might go into effect, say, Monday morning, and the timber companies would cut everything over the weekend."

"It's the same mechanism."

"And the same mindset," Tony said.

"I am shocked, shocked, to find that lobbyists affected the implementation of a law. When have we ever heard of government taking good care of the already-rich?"

"Come on, Derrick. We've heard that cannabis is supposed to be different. Both the plant and the culture surrounding it are immune to capitalism. It's the sacred herb, right?"

Neither of us said anything for a moment.

He said, "It turned into a field day. Anybody with enough capital could buy as many permits as he wanted. In 2017, California issued something over 8,000 permits. Five companies received 730 of them. And this is just going to get worse over time with the centralization of power that always happens as the larger enterprises drive or buy their competitors out of business. It's only been seven years since Colorado legalized pot, and four economic entities control most of the market. Washington and Oregon aren't much better. Nor is Canada, for that matter.

"The whole fee, tax, and regulatory schedule, at both the state and county levels, is so favorable to the already-wealthy that in the first half of 2018, less than 10 percent of the estimated 50,000 growers in California even tried to become aboveground growers. The new rules caused some to quit, and about half were driven back into the unregulated market—the black market, the illegal market, whatever you want to call it—by the new rules.

"A lot of growers couldn't afford the taxes at both the state and county levels. Every government entity wants to wet its beak: 15 percent here, 9.5 percent there. And Humboldt County cultivators have to pay a dollar per square foot of grow canopy. In some municipalities it's up to twenty-five dollars per square foot.

"And then there are the regs. Every bud has to be tracked from clone to sale. Is there any other agricultural product treated this way?

Every tomato tracked? Hell, when you buy a pound of beef at the grocery store it probably came from twenty cows. Or packaging: not only does everything you sell have to be in child-resistant packaging, it also has to be double-packed, with the outside layer opaque so nobody on the street sees a bud. California cannabis alone produces more than a million pieces of single-use plastic per year."

I asked, "And aren't there problems with testing?"

"One of the great things about the Proposition 64 was the intent to get poisons out of the industry. But because it's such a new industry and because it's federally illegal, there weren't real protocols for mass testing, nor were there protocols for tolerance. So, for example, there was a forest fire, and ash from this fire blew into Humboldt County and landed on a lot of people's outdoor grows. Their pot then failed tests for contamination and had to be destroyed. Too bad, so sad, for the growers.

"Or some guy's shatter tested clean, then the lab put it into a container that evidently still had some cleaning solvent in it. Of course it tested dirty after that and had to be destroyed. Tens of thousands of dollars' worth of product.

"There have been cases where bud tested clean, got tested again and failed, then tested again clean, but because it failed one of the tests, it all had to be destroyed. Entire crops."

"And the grower doesn't get paid."

"Not at all. They can easily be out $100,000. A big company can withstand such a loss, but if you're a small grower, you just lost your house. Also, at the start of legalization there were so few testing labs available that there was a four-month backlog. You have to pay up front—thousands and thousands of dollars—for the testing, then wait months and hope you don't fail, so that eventually you can get some money."

I said, "So, instead of barriers to economies of scale, like you had before, you now have barriers to entry, so that starting a grow is too expensive for normal people."

He responded, "Let's contrast the startup costs for an illegal versus legal grow. A decent-sized introductory illegal indoor grow will cost you about $10,000 for everything. Building, lights, pots, soil, plant starts. Then maybe $1,000 per month expenses. An outdoor grow will cost you a couple of hundred bucks for plants and some friend's land, with much lower monthly expenses.

"Let's pretend you're a good person. You don't take water from streams or dump poison on the land. This is, in the best sense, the American Dream. Almost anyone can put together $200 for plants, and a lot of people can save up $10,000—or borrow it from friends and relatives—for a grow room. And you can start your own business. It's cheaper than opening a restaurant or laundromat. It's cheaper than buying even the smallest of houses and becoming a landlord.

"Now, for a legal grow. Let's start with fees to Humboldt County, around $8,000 just to get the paperwork going. And another $10,000 for state licenses. Then you have to pay fees for permits from the California Water Resources Board, Fish and Wildlife, and the county for wastewater and roads. The low end for a grower to enter the legal market would be $35,000 before you even think about any of the expenses associated with the actual growing, like a building or plants. And that's if you do all the work yourself and don't hire a cannabis law consultant to facilitate the process. Realistically you're looking at an absolute minimum of $80,000 to $100,000 for a mom-and-pop grow op to even think about getting into the game.

"And for the record, if you start a legal grow, you can no longer have weapons on your property to defend yourself. Although of course you can hire a private security company. And you also have to pay for the track and trace we mentioned.

"And then the growers have to buy tags for every plant—every plant. These tags cost the grower thousands more.

"But we haven't even talked about the biggest issue, which is the structural changes people have to make to their property. Now, we all know the rural lands in Humboldt have been hammered by industrial logging. And the counties are now requiring that growers who want to get permits also fix problems caused by logging: bad culverts from a former logging company or from a shitty county road construction project. For decades the counties have refused to fix these rural roads, and now they're doing this abatement on the backs of cannabis growers. Oh, and growers have to not just fix them but expand them. Do you love the fact that you live at the far end of a tiny road that winds through wild lands, and you have a small grow to pay your property taxes and put food on the table, but you want to be legal? Well, tough luck, because you have to widen the road so a fire truck can drive to it."

"Presumably complete with pullouts so fire trucks can pass on the road."

"And then there's the 'canopy tax,' where even on outdoor grows you have to pay at least a dollar a square foot on your grow, so if your grow is 10,000 square feet, there's 10K out the door before you plant a seedling. If your crop fails, or gophers eat it, or you get mold—well, tough luck, you're still out the 10K, as well as your labor and your other expenses.

"And because cannabis is illegal at the federal level, you can't get a business loan. Can you imagine any other farmers trying to operate without short-term credit? I have friends even in the aboveground market who are forced to jump from credit card to credit card, and when the credit company finds out they're a small marijuana farm they pull their line of credit. Again, big companies can survive this. Small operations lose the farm.

"And although pot is federally illegal, the feds still stand there with their hands out, demanding taxes. And since we need banking reform surrounding cannabis, there are people who have to walk into the tax office with $100,000 in cash."

"I hope they don't get robbed on the way in."

"The best-case scenario is that the robbery takes place legally, inside the tax buildings.

"And then you've got all those fat cats in Big Canna and all those techbro venture capitalists who've been jumping into the game because they have more money than God at this point. The effect is that these speculators—outsiders with no understanding of or care about traditional cannabis cultures—are coming in and 'bailing out'—read, taking over—these small cannabis farms that have been in these communities for decades.

"The regulated cannabis market has been designed to fail small family farms, and to fail at causing cannabis to be cultivated in ways that are ecologically sane and have even a semblance of sustainability. It's designed to fail at maintaining cannabis culture and at maintaining these cannabis-supported communities. The system was designed by Cannacrats to satisfy the financial needs and desires of the state and overcapitalized corporate techbros.

"Add to this that Humboldt contracted with a private company to use satellites to search for unpermitted cannabis grows. The county just won an award from other counties for its "innovative program" to regulate cannabis by using satellites to police us.

"When they find people out of compliance, the fines can be upwards of ten thousand dollars a day, retroactive. Yes, ten thousand dollars per day. This is just assets forfeiture all over again. The farmstead your back-to-the-lander grandparents worked on through the sixties, paid off in the seventies, and left to your parents and then you, can be lost as quickly as in the midst of Reagan's War on Drugs, because the skid road the county let the logging company build to your house years ago is not up to code. The war on small cannabis farmers hasn't ended at all. It's just taken on a different form. Legalization as it has been put in place is simply Prohibition 2.0. Smarter, sleeker, sneakier, and almost completely unknown to the general public.

"What's interesting to me is that even with all this moneygrubbing, in 2020 Humboldt County lost tax revenue. Only 1 percent, but still down. That's what happens when the county/state drives thousands of growers out of business by these excessive taxes and regulations: sure, they get more direct money, but now they lose taxes they used to get when all those now-out-of-business growers bought their necessities of life, raised their families here. Did they forget the multiplier effect?

"Another interesting thing is that although this has driven a lot of growers out of business, others keep on keeping on. We still have well over eight billion in sales in the traditional—read, illegal—market as compared to three billion in the permitted market. What does that tell us? It tells us that the traditional market is still alive, and their attempts to force people into the regulated market have so far failed.

"Out of the estimated 30,000 growers prior to legalization in Humboldt County, only 450 have applied for licenses—*450*. And only 86 of those are for farms under 5,000 square feet. The majority of permits have gone to those cultivating over 10,000 square feet. The big, rich corporate players, for the most part."

"You talked about barriers to entry before and now for cultivation. Can you talk about them also for distributors?"

"Well, for both cultivation and distribution we'll leave off the risk of prison, in that before, there was a chance you could go to prison for a long time. But as with cultivation, for those willing to take that risk, there were very real possibilities for single mothers to raise their children, for artists to support their work, for people to live the cliché of the American Dream.

"In the old days, the cost to become a distributor was a shitty car that had working taillights, a friend to front you the weed, ten dollars in turkey bags to seal the weed, a blanket to put over the turkey bags, four hundred bucks in gas to get you to Chicago and back, and a friend there who has lots of friends who smoke weed."

"You and I both know people who have done that."

"We both know people who started with nothing and made a living at it."

I said, "I asked a marijuana attorney what it would take to become a legal reseller, and the attorney told me I shouldn't bother going to the state to apply for a permit unless I have $250,000 *cash* on hand."

"And you have to have a fleet of white vans—talk about easy rip-off identifiers—and all sorts of fees for security where you're going to keep the pot."

"As opposed to stashed in your closet in turkey bags."

"Rent for warehouses to store the pot can easily run to $5,000/ month for a small space."

"And when they find you're storing marijuana there they not infrequently triple your rent."

"You have to have all sorts of high-tech surveillance equipment because of the track and trace. You have to pay security companies.

I can see why the attorney told you not to bother unless you have a quarter million in ready cash."

"Which, let's be clear, most normal people don't have."

"We've gone from needing a crappy car, a couple of hundred bucks, and two friends to basically having to be rich enough to drop hundreds of thousands of dollars without blinking."

CHAPTER 9

You've Got Mail

"The internet changed everything," Charlie told me.

Charlie did two tours in Iraq as a Marine, suffering full hearing loss in one ear and a mangled thumb. The hearing loss was from an IED and won him a purple heart, he said, while the mangled thumb "came one day when I sat down too fast, and forgot to take my thumb out of my ass. That one won me the best prize ever." He gestured with his good thumb toward the woman sitting next to him on their couch.

She said, "I was an intake nurse when he came in for his thumb, which had been hit by shrapnel, by the way, not mangled when he sat on it."

He winked and said, "Sitting down on it just slowed the recovery."

She ignored him and continued, "When he walked through the door and I saw him for the first time, I turned to the nurse next to me and said, 'That's the man I'm going to marry.'"

He said, "We went on a couple of dates, and after our tours ended and we got back to the States, we decided I'd go visit her. She lived in Durango, Colorado, and after two tours in Iraq I needed time alone in the wild, so I thought I'd fly out, go hiking and camping for a couple of weeks, then when I got back from the wilderness we'd hang out and get to know each other. We chose that order—backpacking first—because we both wanted to save the best for last.

"But the airline lost my luggage. I still wanted to go camping, and Sheila was kind enough to let me use her backpack and sleeping bag. I spent the next two weeks sleeping enveloped in her pheromones. I never stood a chance. And here we are all these years later. . . . We knew pretty quickly we wanted to make a life together, but we didn't know what that life would look like."

She said, "We've both always loved reading . . ."

He gestured to the walls covered with bookshelves sagging from the weight of the books.

She continued, "But neither of us wanted to go to college."

He said, "Universities weren't as idiotic as they are now, but we both already saw what politically-correct shitshows they were becoming, and after the extended clusterfuck that was the US invasion of Iraq, the last thing either of us needed was another extended clusterfuck. But if we didn't go to college, how would we make a living? Neither of us wanted a life of welcoming people to Walmart, which admittedly would still have been more honest than if we'd gotten degrees in Lit Crit or some other bullshit. What were we going to do? How were we going to pay the rent?"

I asked, "When was this?"

"It was 2006," he said.

She said, "Finally it occurred to us that most of our fellow veteran friends were smoking pot, either to help with their PTSD or for the hell of it, and we could help ourselves and help them by figuring out how to get them access to high-quality, organic weed."

He picked up the story, "We moved here."

To a small town in rural Humboldt. I'm not going to say which one.

"And started to introduce ourselves to our new neighbors."

I asked, "How did you fit in, a couple of veterans in this partly hippy community?"

"Swimmingly," he responded. "There's an interesting mix of lefty perspectives, redneck values, and libertarian ideals out here. And being a marine reinforced what my parents taught me about hard work and discipline, and everybody likes a hard-working neighbor, especially when you help with their crop. It didn't hurt that Sheila makes the world's best strawberry-rhubarb pie as well as the world's best fudge and isn't shy about sharing either of those."

I looked at her, I hoped casually, but I suspect I most closely resembled a dog sitting at your feet as you eat a piece of cheese.

She said, "They're already made. I'll send some home with you."

I thanked her for that entirely unanticipated gift.

She smiled and said, "It also didn't hurt that if their pot was organic, we told them we'd start buying it from them, cash up front."

"Speaking of which," he said, "do you have any pot you'd like for us to move for you?"

When we turned the tape recorder back on,[1] I asked, "How much cash did you start with?"

He said, "By then I was getting a little over $400 per month disability for my hearing loss."

I raised my eyebrows at the low amount.

"The US government has always loved its veterans, in the abstract," he said. "Anyway, we had money for a few months' rent, a small cushion to live on, and enough capital to buy a couple of pounds of outdoor, which we turned over right away to friends around the country who were all-too-happy to get this good shit mailed to their door. We made a few hundred dollars a pound, and plowed everything back into our working capital. Soon we could buy three pounds at a time, then four, then five. And soon some of our neighbors trusted us enough to front us the pot, to be paid a couple of weeks later when we got our cut."

"Was most of this for personal use or resale?"

She said, "Most of the buyers were individuals, but most of the volume was to small-time dealers, people like us making a living in Tampa, Houston, Cleveland, Hartford, or wherever. They'd buy a pound or two per week to distribute to their friends."

"How did—or does—payment work?"

"With personal orders they just send cash to a friend of ours who in exchange for a tiny cut lets us use his address. Then we send the pot. On larger orders the dealer sends 50 percent up front, we send the pot, and they send the rest on receipt. We do this to spread the necessary trust; they have to trust us to send it, and we have to trust them to send the last half.

---

[1] It's a joke! I didn't sell him anything. Maybe because she did all the buying. Again, it's a joke!

"If something goes wrong, on small orders we just replace it. On large orders we split the loss with the recipient."

"What can go wrong?"

"The most common loss is theft somewhere in the mails. We've had enough stuff disappear in the San Francisco sorting facility to presume there's a ring of thieves—or many independent thieves, or maybe a single really busy one—opening packages of the right size and weight, then stealing the ones worth money."

I told them about the other person I interviewed who also told me about thieves in the San Francisco sorting facility, then asked, "Do customers ever rip you off?"

"Not often," he said. "Especially not the personal customers, who are almost always our brothers and sisters from the military. We've literally been to war together. We'd sooner die than steal from each other."

She laughed and said, "Not that everyone who was in the military—or even our units—is a good person. We're just talking about the ones we stayed in contact with."

He continued, "Some of the dealers, however, are not so honorable. Again, we'd die for the ones we know, so we'll gladly front them some pot. But it gets hard when you move beyond your friends to their friends and then theirs, and then the friends of those people, and some guy's cousin, and so on.

"Some of them are just fuckups. They pay half up-front for their first pound of weed, receive it, smoke it all with their friends, don't have any money to pay us the rest, then are somehow surprised when we won't sell them another pound, or worse, front it to them altogether.

"Much worse are the social engineers. We always start small with new customers—a pound, then a couple of pounds—and slowly work our way up as we grow to trust each other. And if we keep it up, it's sustainable and money-making for both us and them. But it has happened, I think twice now, that someone has built up that trust so they can make a big score. The worst was some guy who became our best customer for a while, building to 20K of pot per week, out of which we'd make a couple of thousand. Then he bumped it up to 40K and said he needed it in a hurry to resell to a big buyer. He'd been consistent enough that we sent it as soon as we got the tracking number on his envelope of cash. But the envelope arrived empty except for a note that said, 'Thanks for the free pot, suckers. It's been nice ripping you off.'"

"Did that make you want to use any of your Marine training on him?"

"Hell, yeah. We fantasized regularly about having a unit reunion in Gainesville, Florida, to kick some ass."

"Why didn't you?"

"Two reasons. One is we presumed he had—like us—used a drop house, so we'd have been busting in on an innocent person, and as much as we wanted to get our own back, we had no interest in harming an innocent person in the hope this person would tell us how to find him. I've already hurt enough bystanders in my life. I don't want to do it anymore.

"And also, it's just not who we are. I mean, we've taken our turns armed in outdoor grows just before harvest, and we'd do whatever we needed to do, but like locks on doors, these patrols are mainly to keep honest people honest. I've been in firefights before, and I'm not eager to be in any more, especially over money."

She said, "These thefts make you understand, though, how and why criminal gangs so often end up so violent. If you run a shoe store, the police at the very least provide a deterrent to robbery. When you're growing or selling marijuana, you cannot turn to the police, and the only deterrents you now have besides good relationships with your neighbors are you and your weapons."

I said, "When I taught creative writing at a supermax, one of my students had been in prison since the seventies. He'd been a marijuana dealer, and someone tried to rob him. He shot and killed the guy, got sentenced to seven to life, and was still in thirty years later. Had he run a shoe store, he wouldn't even have been arrested."

"We are aware of that sort of difference every single day," he said.

"What," I asked, "is the worst thing that's ever happened to your business?"

A look passed between them, one I didn't understand, before she slightly nodded, and then he said, "The time Russian hackers stole $70,000."

"But before we can tell you about that, we have to talk about the internet," she said. "And before we can talk about that, we have to talk about how streaky this business can be. To make the math easy, let's ignore the small buyers, and say we're selling four pounds every two weeks to each of three dealers, at $250 profit per pound. That's $1,500/week profit. We're making bank. Then let's say one of them quits the business for reasons unknown to us. She could have set herself a limit on how much money she wanted to make and met it, so retired. She could have been threatened by another dealer, so quit. She could have gotten one too many scares of cops driving by her home, so quit. She might be in the midst of a divorce, or might have been in a horrible car wreck. For security reasons we usually don't know much about the ones who weren't already our friends. And sometimes we'll work with people for years and then never hear from them again. Let's say you lose two customers in quick succession, and now you're down to $500/week profit. That—along with Charlie's disability payments—is enough to live on. Then you lose three packages in a row to theft or just USPS mistakes—this happens maybe a half to 1 percent of the time, where a package gets ripped apart by machinery, or is misdelivered, or something—which means you just lost twelve pounds of pot. Let's say this pot was top quality indoor, which right now costs you $2,500/lb. You just lost $30,000, or sixty weeks' worth of profit.

"And then the last dealer you've got decides she wants to focus on getting a law degree, and, except for a friend or two on the side, won't have time to sell pot anymore, so her four pounds every two weeks cuts back to a pound every two months.

"You now have essentially no income.

"And how do you find more dealers? It's like fishing. You have to keep your line in the water, but doing so is no guarantee you'll catch any keepers."

He said, "That's how things were—and had been for about a year—when one night Sheila literally saved the homestead. She's always been a late-night person, and I kept military hours long before I joined the military, so one night she came in and woke me at about two, saying, 'Everything's going to be okay.'"

She said, "I'd been noodling on the internet, looking up random stuff like 'how long do snapping turtles live' when it occurred to me to search for 'online drug market.' I learned about one called Silk Road. Not the one in history. The one online."

I'd heard of it.

She continued, "I knew nothing about this and nothing about computers. I could send emails to my parents, look up stuff on recipes.com, and that's about it. Silk Road was, I learned, on something called the dark web. Everything I knew about the dark web I'd learned from watching BBC mysteries, with scary tales of hackers blackmailing internet users and conmen pushing phony pharmaceuticals from India that killed people who bought unprescribed sleeping pills.

"The reality was simpler and less scary. The dark web was, to my limited understanding, just a part of the internet you could only access through a special 'Tor' browser. How this browser works is beyond me. The point is that it's a way to be on the internet anonymously."

I responded, "Which is, given how Facebook, Google, and other companies mercilessly data-mine, track, and censor us, not a bad thing even if you aren't doing anything illegal."

"No doubt," he said.

She continued, "So I downloaded and installed Tor, which was basically plug-and-play, then fairly quickly found Silk Road, made an account, and had my mind blown. It was a bazaar where thousands of sellers openly sold almost every drug imaginable—as well as things like fake IDs and no-ID-required foreign bank accounts—to scores of thousands of buyers worldwide. It was the strangest thing to see eBay-style offerings for cocaine, heroin, LSD, steroids, prescription drugs from India, and on and on."

I asked, "How did you feel about those drugs being so easily available?"

"You mean, apart from flabbergasted?" she responded. "I laughed so loud I startled our cat. I couldn't stop laughing at the absurdity of it.

But beyond that, Charlie and I pretty much draw the line at weed and mushrooms. We've both seen what heroin, meth, and coke can do to people."

"And steroids," he added.

She nodded. "So no, I'm not keen on it. That said, if society is going to have people who are addicted to drugs, I'd think it would be safer for all concerned—including bystanders—to have it available by mail order rather than in person. By mail you don't have to worry about armed robberies or violent turf wars. Can you imagine *The Wire* if all the drug deals were online? Most of those poor kids would be alive."

He said, "Of course the show would be pretty boring."

She said, "And then I saw the category *Cannabis*. I thought, this is it. I went in and woke up Charlie, then said, 'We're not going to lose our home.'"

"When was this?" I asked.

"Early 2012," she said. "We got up on Silk Road pretty quick, and then we got lucky. There were lots of vendors who literally never sold anything, but we got a few sales right away, got great reviews for our customer service and our pot, which led to more sales, which led to more good reviews, which led to even more sales. It felt good to be making a steady living, and it also felt good to be part of the first online drug marketplace, at least for the marijuana part. It felt like we were making history."

"How did sales work?"

"Part of the brilliance of Silk Road was their escrow system that made it so buyer and seller didn't have to trust each other. If you wanted to buy some weed from me, you deposited money."

"How?" I asked.

"I'd never heard of bitcoin before I signed up for Silk Road. I still don't know how it works. I just know it's 'cryptocurrency'—and I don't how that works either—which means it's semi-anonymous online money."

Charlie said, "We look at bitcoin kind of the way we look at cars or computers. Most of us don't know how they work. We just want them to 'go' when we step on the gas or push a button. Or for that matter like we look at sex. I don't think most of us know the precise biochemical mechanics . . ."

"I do," Sheila said.

"But we still like to do it."

"So you're saying bitcoin is like sex," I said.

He answered, "I wouldn't go that far."

"*Anyway*," she said. "You buy some bitcoin and deposit it at Silk Road, then make your purchase. The bitcoin leaves your account but doesn't go into my account until you mark the item as having been received. Then there were various conflict-resolution protocols for anything that might go wrong.

"Silk Road would take a small commission on every sale. They sold huge volumes, and made tons of money."

Charlie said, "It didn't hurt their bank accounts that bitcoin went up."

"It didn't hurt ours, either," she said, then added fondly, "Ah, bitcoin. When we started selling weed on Silk Road a bitcoin was worth about $5. So an ounce of pot that went for $200 would be 40 bitcoins."

He commented, "If we would've known then that bitcoin was going to rise to $50,000 and held onto them, that would have been $2,000,000 per ounce of pot."

"But of course, we didn't know that," she said. "For all we knew bitcoin could go to zero and we'd have been giving away the pot. Plus, we needed cash to buy the pot we sold, so we generally turned the bitcoins over as fast as we could."

"How did you sell the bitcoins?" I asked.

She answered, "Bitcoin wasn't as common as it is now, so to facilitate commerce on Silk Road several vendors bought your bitcoin for just under par and sent you cash. I'm not sure how they then unloaded their bitcoins to the site's buyers, but obviously that's what they were doing."

Charlie said, "Selling bitcoin off the site was a nightmare. It was all completely unregulated and many or most of the exchanges were scams. You sent in bitcoins to sell, and they stole them."

"Either that or Russian hackers stole them."

"One night Sheila woke me about three in the morning, crying, 'They're stealing all our money.' We'd been able to make a few trades on one of the exchanges without getting ripped off, so we went to convert all our bitcoin to cash. We sent everything to one exchange—$70,000—and tried to sell it. A couple of hours later our account had been drained."

"How did you know it was Russian hackers?"

"Theft of bitcoin was so common," he said, "that there sprang up a category of hackers who acted essentially as bounty hunters, or treasure seekers. They would track down your stolen bitcoin in exchange for some percentage of what was taken. There was no risk, so we tried it. The bounty hunter was able to track it to Russia, but the thieves confused the trail enough that he—presuming it was a he—lost it."

She said, "We lost nearly everything we'd worked for over that."

He responded, "I'm surprised bitcoin survived the rampant thefts. *Disgrace* is too weak a word to describe the early bitcoin markets. It really stinks when the bitcoin venders on an illegal drug site on the dark market were less dishonest than the aboveground bitcoin exchanges. If we would have had any alternative currency, we would have taken it, and if we would have had an alternative way of selling weed, we would have quit the online markets altogether. But we didn't have a choice."

She said, "Fortunately there arose some decentralized marketplaces where you could exchange bitcoin for cash in person."

"How'd that work?"

Charlie and Sheila exchanged another look, then he said, "I'd love to tell you, but it's kind of an arms race between people like us trying to come up with ways to anonymously convert bitcoin to cash and various governments trying to figure out who we are. We've had to become really creative, and cagey. And this is highly illegal, so, as the saying goes, if I told you I'd have to—"

She cut him off, and finished by saying, "Send you home without pie or fudge."

I put my fingers together and zipped my lips.

He said, "In some ways it played to our favor that we had trouble selling bitcoin, in that when it started going up, we made a fair amount of money. We had all these coins we'd acquired at $5 each, and we were excited when the price went to $10, and then $15, and then $20, and on up."

She said, "That took some of the sting out of the theft of $70,000. We'd made that much on bitcoin going up."

"Of course," he added, "If we want to look at this as glass half-empty, we could also say that the $70,000 the hackers stole would by now be worth scores of millions."

She said, "I'd rather not think about it that way. I'd rather not think about it at all."

"I have a bitcoin story," I said. "I like betting on sports. I'm not good at it, but the bets are small enough that I usually only lose a hundred or so dollars a year. It's cheap entertainment. When bitcoin was $100, I deposited one bitcoin at a betting site. Over the next couple of years, I lost about .3 bitcoin betting, but meanwhile the price had risen to $10,000, so now I had .7 bitcoin worth $7,000. Then someone stole 90 percent of what I had in there—I later learned this website was notorious for this, so it was probably an inside job—leaving me with about $700. I got confused as to whether I lost $6,300 on this deal or made $600 on my original investment. I didn't know whether to be sad, glad, or wind my watch."

They laughed, and he said, "We wished we would have cashed out when it briefly got almost to $20K, but again, we don't know the future, and after that it all crashed again down to a couple of thousand. We thought it might all go to zero. I didn't understand any of it."

She said, "And now of course it's over $50K."

"How long did you last at Silk Road?" I asked.

He said, "In 2013, Silk Road was seized by the feds, and its founder was arrested and eventually sentenced to multiple life terms for drug trafficking, money laundering, and so on. Several of the vendors were arrested, too."

"Including one guy," Sheila said, "who had his vendor-name on his vanity license plates, and when they arrested him, he had an apartment full of shirts with his logo on them."

"By then," Charlie continued, "the idea of online drug markets was in the public, and stores were springing up all over: Black Market Reloaded. Silk Road 2. Silk Road 3. Alpha Bay. Dream. Empire. Wall Street Market. The Cannabis Growers Market Collective, which only allowed weed and shrooms. So many others.

"Some, like Alpha Bay, were busted and their owners arrested. Some, like Black Market Reloaded, lasted for a while, then when the owner had made a pile, declared an orderly closure, and the owner rode off into the sunset. Others, like Dream and Silk Road 2, were what are called exit scams. That's where the market builds up confidence by running for several months or maybe a year, then suddenly shuts down and steals all the buyers' and venders' bitcoins. The largest exit scam we know of was Empire Market, which took about $30 million in bitcoin."

She said, "To prevent that risk, these days a lot of online market-places don't require individuals to deposit at the market, but run more like eBay, where you keep your money in your own off-site account and transfer the bitcoin only when you make a purchase. After escrow, it goes directly to the vendor's offsite account. The only money that could be stolen by the marketplace is what's in escrow."

I said, "You began by saying that the internet changed everything. How precisely has everything changed?"

He said, "The other day I talked to an old-timer who has been selling since the late seventies. He's mainly retired, but keeps his hand in. He doesn't do anything online. He told me that in the old days, connections were everything. If you live in northern California, it doesn't do you any good to be the best grower in the world if you don't know someone who knows someone who knows someone who sells in Little Rock, Arkansas. And likewise, someone can be the best and most honest dealer in Vicksburg, Mississippi, but that doesn't do him—"

"Or her—" Sheila said

"—any good if he, or she, doesn't know someone who knows someone who knows someone here in northern California who can provide some good pot. This was why in the old days it was worth it to put twenty pounds of pot in sealed containers in the trunk of your beat-up Chevy and drive to Detroit to meet with a friend of a friend, and this was why it was worth it for people from Boston to drive to northern California every few months with $100,000 in cash to pick up pot and reconnect with old friends."

"These days," she said, "a dealer in Atlanta can buy some bitcoin, fire up the Tor browser, and have five pounds of pot on its way by the next morning. Or someone in Manhattan can do the same and buy an ounce of her favorite strain for personal use to help her deal with the trauma of living in New York City."

I said, "So it's kind of like everything on the internet. With a few clicks I can buy anything from frozen waffles to a first edition of *Scaramouche*, to recycled wood flooring."

He said, "And you can do it all in your pajamas."

She said, "Maybe that will someday be considered the crowning achievement of the internet: it allows people to buy top quality weed sitting on the couch wearing pajamas."

CHAPTER 10

Perseverance

I spoke again with Tony. Because of Covid, we spoke over Skype. I hadn't seen him in months and was surprised at his full beard.

I asked, "If they made you czar of all things marijuana on either the state or national level, how would you change the way legalization has taken place to help the cottage industry, consumers, and the natural world?"

He responded, "The first thing I'd do is stop listening to Big Canna when making regulations. I'd go directly to traditional cannabis communities and have meaningful conversations. I'd really listen to them, not create the sort of dog and pony show Newsom and others put us through. Not the phony public input schemes we're all so familiar with.

"Next, I wouldn't view all regulation through the lens of revenue. Currently, revenue is the driving force. Not communities, and certainly not wild nature.

"Third, I'd craft policies that aim toward regenerating the natural world.

"In terms of actual rules, I would—pending conversations with those in the cottage industry—remove the heavy taxes and obscene licensing fees for small cultivators, packagers, and sellers and make them more in line with other agricultural ventures. And I would attempt to get all of the agencies on the same page, so growers would only need to deal with one bureaucracy instead of separately with the water board, Fish and Game, public health, department of agriculture, local planning, and on and on.

"I'd also rein in planning departments. I wanted to put in a hoop house to grow tomatoes—real tomatoes, not wink-wink tomatoes—and even though it didn't have electricity or plumbing—literally a hoop greenhouse—I was told I had to hire an engineer and then pay hundreds of dollars for a permit. For tomatoes!

"It's far worse for cannabis growers. The planning department in this county has been given police-like authority over cultivators, which it uses to shake them down for thousands of dollars. If I were marijuana czar, I'd return the planning department to planning and remove their ability to enforce or fine.

"One reason I keep hammering this is that the Eye in the Sky surveillance program I mentioned the last time we talked is part of the planning department. Think about that: the county planning department using satellite technology provided by a private corporation to surveil its residents from outer space. Yeah, that's happening, and taxpayers are funding it.

"And the whole point is to make money. It's certainly not to protect the environment—which should frankly be a primary purpose of any planning department. They certainly aren't surveilling Big Ag and the timber industry. At the same time that they're forcing people who live within city limits to get permits before they can put in a hoop house, and at the same time that they're spying on us from outer space, they're granting permits for large cultivators living off-grid to run diesel generators for electric lighting *for outdoor grows*. Worse, on outdoor grows next to public lands with old growth forests and endangered spotted owl habitat. This is completely insane.

"If you're a small grower, you pay huge fees for a tiny grow house, but if you've got the capital, they'll let you destroy habitat for endangered species—especially nocturnal species—through light and noise pollution as well as, of course, the greenhouse gases and other air pollution from the diesel generators. If I were in charge, I'd stop that in a hot minute.

"The next thing I'd do is ban all large-scale indoor growing for recreational marijuana. I'm not talking about banning people's personal closet grows, or even small cottage scenes. But it's ridiculous, even with new technologies like LEDs, that we allow square-block industrial grows for the recreational market. It's too much strain on the grid, and it shows how little we as a society care about global warming or conserving energy in general. Half of the growth in electricity demand in Colorado between 2012 and 2014 was from indoor grows. New grows coming online in Portland, Oregon, caused a half-dozen power outages in 2015. Indoor weed already consumes 1 percent of the electricity in the United States—3 percent in California—and experts predict that within a few years marijuana industry use will exceed that of data centers.

"Sure, some medical marijuana needs to be grown indoors for consistency of specific strengths and mixes of THC and other cannabinoids—but just to get high there's no reason people can't smoke outdoor weed.

"Some of the problem is cultural, in that consumers have a fetish for indoor, in part because it often looks more uniform with tighter, smoother buds. It's like when we go to the grocery store and won't buy organic fruit because of tiny blemishes. Instead, we pick the beautiful, yet waxy and toxic, fruit. The fetish for indoor weed is really a fetish for the industrial.

"My next policy recommendation would depend on how much power I had. If it's only a fair amount, I would reinstate the five-year moratorium on large grows in California that was in the proposition we passed. If I had more power, I would institute a permanent ban on large-scale grows, so you can have a maximum of one permit per person and one acre per permit.

"The questions would be: How do you protect the carrying capacity of the natural landscape, and how do you protect the conscious cottage growers? And another question would be: Now that the various states have fucked over small growers, how do we fairly fix problems Big Canna and the Cannacrats created? I don't care about Big Canna as such, since Big Canna doesn't hesitate to screw small growers out of their livelihoods—as Big Ag doesn't hesitate to screw over family farmers, as Big Box Stores don't hesitate to screw over local businesses, as chain bookstores don't hesitate to screw over local bookstores, and as

Amazon doesn't hesitate to screw over everyone—but Big Canna does employ people, so we'd need to phase out Big Canna in a way that was fair to their employees.

"The point is that I would remove the incentives for large-scale farming, the disincentives for small-scale farming, and certainly remove the barriers to entry with which small cultivators struggle.

"Currently, counties are allowed to ban cannabis cultivation, which mainly drives people back into the unregulated market where there's no environmental oversight. I'd want to revisit the idea of local bans. We don't locally ban wineries, do we? When was the last time some locality banned tomato farms? The only reason cannabis farms are banned is because we still have a prohibitionist mindset."

He thought a moment, then said, "Electric companies give their commercial rate to cannabis businesses, which incentivizes indoor production. I would eliminate that.

"I would address the terrible overpackaging problem, and the production of plastic waste, including that in vape pens and oil cartridges. Millions of oil cartridges are destined to end up in waterways and in fish and other wildlife, just like the rest of our garbage. There's no recycling mandate in this industry. I would change that the moment I became czar. I would also curtail or eliminate synthetic pesticides and curtail or eliminate water withdrawal from streams that are critical habitat for critters. Much of the industry is an environmental nightmare, and that's not acceptable.

"And here I come to maybe my most unpopular perspective. If I were a czar for marijuana at the federal level, I would eliminate state bans on marijuana cultivation and then over time institute fairly generous caps on how much each state could produce. Cannabis is such a beautifully adaptable plant—called weed, remember—that there's no reason each bioregion couldn't begin to develop its own cannabis culture.

"The question about cannabis—and about everything else, really—is how much is enough? In 2017, California produced 14 million pounds of cannabis. Californians consumed about 2.5 million pounds, so we produced more than five times what we consumed, which means the pot is going elsewhere—and that elsewhere might possibly grow cannabis with less of an ecological footprint than what's happening here."

I said, "Of course with this you're not just talking about cannabis."

"Absolutely not. The global economy is a disaster for the natural world, and for poor humans the world over. And the more it globalizes, the more it wrecks local economies. We need to be supporting local economies, whether those economies are local food networks, local cannabis networks, you name it."

I asked, "Part of the point of this book has been that legalization has harmed cannabis culture and the cottage industry, especially in northern California. Wouldn't stopping regional exports do even more harm?"

He responded, "I wouldn't want to stop regional exports as such. I just don't think we can have a cottage industry producing high-quality cannabis with a minimal ecological footprint while we also have an infinitely expanding cannabis industry."

I said, "Just like we can't have any infinitely expanding industry on a finite planet."

"Exactly. I obviously have no interest in destroying the cottage industry, which legalization is doing wherever it's currently enacted. But if we're going to survive—*we* as in human beings on a living planet—we have to recognize there are limits. And we need to start thinking ecologically and bioregionally. That's all I'm saying. Nobody needs a ten-acre grow to survive economically. One acre, sure. Ten acres, no."

He paused, stroked his beard, then said, "Now I'll get back to saying things that won't make the cottage growers hate me. Not only do we need to stop counties shaking down small growers, we need to create programs that can help traditional cultivators get into compliance. Currently, it's simply the stick, right? You need to pay all this money upfront, and then if you do something wrong, we fine you thousands of dollars per day. How about giving them assistance on the ground, through consultations, advice, access to professionals who can help them fix problems like those caused by the timber industry, and so on. The real question is not how do we force current landowners to fix problems caused by prior landowners but how do we as a society fix problems caused by destructive prior land uses?

"The road systems in these communities are horrible: they're old logging roads. And no one has the money to fix them. The problem with having cannabis growers pay for them is that they didn't create these problems in the first place. Honestly it should be the timber companies and other extractive industries that fix these problems."

"But we know that will never happen."

"Never," he said. Then, "If I were in charge of marijuana, I would also bring in labor standards, which are not well-developed right now in either the aboveground or belowground industries. I would provide cultivators with expertise in developing worker safety and training programs."

I said, "A couple of times you've mentioned one permit per person. How would you enforce that? I'm thinking, for example, of the Homestead Act, where individuals were supposed to get land from the government. But speculators would go to bars, round up a bunch of drunk people, have them sign papers, and before you knew it the rich guy had title to twenty square miles."

Tony said, "We'd have to put in strict penalties against that and enforce them. I don't have an answer beyond that, since that's not so much a cannabis problem but a larger problem of corruption as well as the government often creating laws that, intentionally or not, have loopholes through which wealthy people can drive trucks full of cash. It's not just the Homestead Act. It's every act like that. It's equity programs, where permits are supposed to be preferentially given to members of minority groups, but not infrequently white people with money find a random brown person to pretend to go into business with in order to get those advantages. It's also precisely the whole marijuana legalization fiasco.

"But it's not just governments. It's also people. Remember the rented Prop 215 cards? People are going to try to game the system, so whoever is charged with enforcement would have to figure out ways to stay one step ahead of the thieves, more politely called speculators.

"Just today I was looking at something on YouTube, and a commercial came on that featured a white, conservative-looking, church-going-type guy telling me to invest in cannabis: 'You don't have to smoke it,' he said, 'for it to be a good investment.'

"So really the question is the same one faced by family farmers of all types, and local shop owners, and bookstore owners, and members of every other cottage industry—which is how do we keep the rich speculators out? How do we keep them from destroying our livelihoods?"

"It's a question people have been trying to answer since the time of the guilds, certainly since the Luddites."

"And we need to keep living our way into answers that will stop them," he said.

I asked, "You keep talking about wanting to get rid of the fees and taxes on small growers. But a lot of counties and even states are trying to balance their budgets on cannabis revenues, including spending the money on social programs. Wouldn't your ideas literally take food out of children's mouths?"

He responded, "First, I'm not suggesting getting rid of taxes altogether. Instead of fees and square-footage taxes that have to be paid before you're able to sell anything, I don't think most growers would find a simple excise or sales tax on the final product objectionable.

"Next, recall that county income in Humboldt went down because of these fees, and because of the multiplier effect. When people have money, they spend it at the local furniture store, the local bookstore, local restaurants."

"I know a single mother," I said, "who has been the sole employee—half-time—of a small farmer for ten years. It's been her sole income. Twenty dollars an hour under the table hasn't made her wealthy, but it's kept her off welfare and in a small house. And all of that money has gone right back into the community for food, clothing, school supplies. She spends the rest of her time raising her daughter."

"Healthy traditional cannabis communities enable people to stay in these rural communities, which means these communities will have money for schools and social services.

"The last few summers, before and as legalization started to kick in, I spent time in a small town on the Lost Coast called Petrolia. It's a back-to-the-land community with cannabis central to the local economy. There are a lot of older people in the area who want to stay on their land—one of the most beautiful spots on Earth. They're not working in the regular economy. And young people come in to grow cannabis and to trim. They rent local people's land. And because these young people can make a living, many of them stay, and they raise children there. The money they make pays into the local economy. The kids go to the local schools. With legalization, these small-scale traditional cultivators are getting priced out of the market because they can't afford the taxes and fees. And when these farms shut down the young people leave—"

"Same as in Iowa," I said.

"Same as in the Rust Belt. Same as anywhere the economy gets gutted. So then the teachers are no longer needed because there aren't as many kids. Now the teachers can no longer afford to live there. They move away. And the old people no longer get the marijuana rent on their land. Some have to move out entirely. It's a cascading failure of the community.

"Because of the way legalization has played out, communities are basically disappearing in rural parts of the Emerald Triangle. And many of the people who are leaving are the ones you don't want leaving: the back-to-the-landers, the ones who are ecologically conscious, the ones who were rehabilitating the landscapes on their properties.

"And the timber companies and land speculators are moving back in. Everybody who lives in these places understands this."

I said, "When it comes to Walmart, Amazon, or for that matter prisons, government officials at every level from local to national understand all this. It's one reason they do away with property taxes and give all sorts of other financial breaks to these huge corporations on the understanding that the governments will make their money back through the employees who live there."

Tony responded, "But when it comes to pot, they have their hands out up front, even though they can make more money down the line."

He stopped, looked aside, stroked his beard again, then said, "And we haven't even touched on indigenous people and their role in crafting regulations and having power to make land-use decisions over cannabis. Just down the road from my house is Yurok land. They are river people. The feds gave them only a small strip, but their traditional land goes all up and down the river. Most of that land is long-since privatized. Some of that land is used for growing cannabis.

"How do we respect the rights of First Nations when it comes to cannabis? Indigenous people themselves are split on it. It's much like casinos. Some people are like, 'Bring it on. We need the money.' Others say, 'We have enough problems. We don't need the problems brought by gambling/cannabis.' This is something we don't talk about enough in the Emerald Triangle, and something that desperately needs to be part of the discussion."

"In our last conversation, you called legalization Prohibition 2.0. Can you expand on that?"

"Back when marijuana was illegal, California had CAMP, the Campaign Against Marijuana Planting, which was a militarized police force aimed at eradicating marijuana cultivation. Not so many people know this, but the government is still using militarized police forces to eradicate marijuana. The National Guard. And it's not on public lands. It's illegal grows on private lands. Or at this point the more accurate term is 'unpermitted grows.' And each summer the sheriff in Humboldt County requests the military fly over to find unpermitted grows. Not just big grows. Little grows too. Anyone trying to get out from under the county shaking them down for permits.

"The California Bureau of Cannabis Control has created a special branch of law enforcement—none of this was in Prop 64 as it was passed, nor has it really been vetted by the public—and is asking lawmakers to allow them to create a ninety-member tactical SWAT squad. *To enforce failures to get permits.* Cannabis is no longer illegal in California. This is not an armed police force to stop murders or home invasions. This is not a police force to interdict illegal drugs like heroin, or even as cannabis used to be. It's not about busting Walter White and his meth lab. This is about an armed police force going after people who have failed or refused to hand over large amounts of money to get permits. This is like sending armed police after people who are growing tomatoes without permits.

"This is an armed police force to impose the dictates of Big Canna and the Cannacrats, to put the fear of God—or cops—back into the traditional cannabis growers and distributors.

"They never acknowledge that this is about generating profit for Big Canna. The justification these days is environmental and consumer protection. But when did they ever send armed police out to stop clearcutting?

"It's all the prohibitionist mindset with the added twist of making it so states can wet their beaks on this formerly untapped revenue stream.

"Here's a quote by the president of the California Association of Criminal Investigators, the union representing employees who will be part of this bureau: 'Knowing firsthand how rampant the unlicensed and credible criminal cannabis activity is in the state, there is a definite need for additional police officers to assist in the control and enforcement of the laws set forth by legislators and by propositions enacted by citizens of California.'[1] Again, this is about unlicensed growers, not murderers. Or for that matter, polluters who happen to be licensed. If I were the marijuana czar, I would stop that shit in a heartbeat. Sure, we need enforcement of environmental regulations, but I wouldn't use the power of the state to force small growers out of business."

He stopped, took a drink of water, and said, "If I were czar, I would also overhaul the relationship between banking and the cannabis industry. If you recall, last time we talked about how cannabis cultivators can't get crop or other short-term loans. I would make it so cannabis businesses can access banking services, savings accounts, and lines of credit and make it so they can't be discriminated against simply for being in that industry."

I said, "Given what happened to the Luddites; given what's been happening with family farms from the fifties through the nineties until

---

[1] Andrew Sheeler, "California wants to hire more cannabis cops to get a handle on black market marijuana," *Sacramento Bee*, June 2, 2020.

today; given what happened with the organic standards the US government passed in the nineties that had the same effects as marijuana legalization, in that organic farmers had to go through processes they couldn't afford, but rich companies could, driving honest-to-goodness organic farmers out of business—what would you do?

"In other words, everything in this conversation so far has presumed you are the marijuana czar and also that you are bulletproof. But given current political and economic reality, given the centralization that takes place in capitalism, what would you suggest people do?"

"The first thing I'd suggest has to do with appellations."

"Like the mountains? How does West Virginia fit in?"

He didn't laugh, which was good because I wasn't making a joke. I had no idea what he was saying, nor, evidently, how to spell it.

He said, "Appellations are legally defined and protected geographical indicators. We most often hear about these for wine, and sometimes for cheese. For example, champagne comes from one region in France. No other region should be allowed to label their product *champagne*. When you buy *champagne*, you know it deserves the name because of the soil the plants were grown in, the air they breathed. The same is true for some cheeses. Parmigiano Reggiano is a designated name for a specific cheese made using specific processes in a specific part of Italy. In the European Union, no other cheese can be called Parmesan. In the United States other cheeses can be called Parmesan, but none can be called Parmigiano Reggiano."

"How would that work with cannabis?"

"The Emerald Triangle is famous worldwide for growing the best marijuana in the world. But right now, someone could grow marijuana in a greenhouse in Santa Barbara and call it Emerald Triangle Bud. The name is legally meaningless.

"The appellation program would be designed to indicate where the marijuana is grown, how it's grown, and its quality. Then the consumer could make educated choices, just like consumers can currently make educated choices about whether to buy real champagne or Freixenet sparkling plonk, whether to buy real Parmigiano Reggiano or some of the American brands of 'parmesan cheese' that contain no parmesan whatsoever and up to 8 or 9 percent wood pulp.

"This protects both consumer and producer.

"In this case it would give traditional cannabis growers a way to market their product that not only protects the integrity of the cannabis but also allows them to survive by producing small-scale, beautiful cannabis.

"I would love to see watershed-based appellations showing that this or that bud was grown not just in the Emerald Triangle but on the Van Duzen River just above where it runs into the Eel River. And not only that but grown organically outdoors without harming salmon. And not only that but specific strains.

"This model is being developed right now in Humboldt and Mendocino counties by a group called the Origins Council.[2] This is something everyone can participate in. But in the end, will governments listen to small growers and to consumers, or will Big Canna turn this into a shell of what it could be?

"We don't know. But it's an example of what's possible—and has been done elsewhere—to protect artisans from big corporations.

"I also think more and more growers should look into local cooperatives. To cultivate even one acre requires farm equipment, space to properly dry the materials, and so on. That can be expensive, and there's no reason some of that equipment and space can't be shared.

"And people need to be politically-engaged, especially on the local level. You've got to attend the planning commission meetings. You've got to attend the board of supervisors' meetings. Don't get me wrong. I'm not all rah-rah about the almost-entirely-corrupt political process in this country, but when it comes to smaller communities like mine, if you get fifty people to show up at a meeting of local government, it can make a difference.

"We also need to work hard on consumer education. If people are buying weed and know nothing about the company or how it's grown and can't name where it's grown, we've got problems."

---

[2] https://originscouncil.org/.

"We can make," I said, "the same argument about tomatoes, canta-loupes, and t-shirts."

"I wish I was more optimistic. But when I started researching can-nabis and the environment, I would talk to students about pesticides on their weed. I'd ask how well they know their dealer. Usually, not well. And do you know where your dealer gets weed? Usually, they didn't care. They just wanted good, stinky pot. These were students at liberal Humboldt State University, buying organic pro-duce at the co-op, talking nonstop about the importance of organic, sustainable agriculture but buying chemical-laden weed, grown God-knows-where."

I asked, "Wouldn't consumer education be impossible for legal rea-sons in an unregulated or illegal market? There has to be firewalls at every part of the process. Let's say you're in Kentucky. You know your dealer, but you have to take the dealer's word that the pot is organic. You can't know the farmer. You can't tour the farm."

"My response—and this is going to piss off my neighbors again—would be that the person in Kentucky should stop buying California weed and find a local grower. Of course, in the current environment that isn't possible. Which is one reason weed needs to be legalized, with caps on grow size. Then none of this would be a problem."

"What else do you suggest people do politically and socially?"

"No matter how much I promote people buying local weed, I fully recognize that's not a real solution."

I said, "That's like talking about sustainability within civilization. Within this larger unsustainable superstructure there are no real solu-tions. Which doesn't mean we can't make things less bad."

"That's one reason among many I don't have much faith in the political system. So I'm not a fan of going to legislators in the capitol and lobbying for this or that. As opposed to locally. Having said that, I do think voter initiatives can be helpful. It worked for Prop 215. And also, having said that, I do think people need to try to be involved in at least learning the shape legislation might be taking at state and federal levels. Those laws could be more or less restrictive and could be more or less friendly to cottage industries. And if governments are going to destroy cottage industries, create a shitstorm. Because otherwise legislators will only listen to Big Canna."

"What would you like to say to the old-school environmentally-conscious cannabis cultivators who are disheartened by how legalization has played out?"

"I would say, keep on keeping on. You survived Prohibition, and you will survive Prohibition 2.0. Illegal grows were an act of civil disobedience in the seventies, and they are an act of resistance now. I know the deck is stacked against you, but that has always been the case.

"Most of the small-scale growers I've spoken with who are in the regulated market are also in the traditional market. They can't survive without the underground.

"I have good friends who are remaining in the traditional market because they can't afford the licensing fees, but who are following the legal environmental standards because it's the right thing to do. And many are going beyond those environmental standards.

"So what I would say to those old-school cannabis cultivators who have been doing this for decades is: If you want, stay unregulated. If you can hide from the Eye in the Sky, do it. But don't harm salmon. Don't harm martens. And don't poison consumers.

"And never forget to celebrate this wonderful plant. It's a gift, and we've been misusing this gift, both by declaring it to be evil through reefer madness and by treating it purely as a means to make money. Both of those approaches are wrong and disrespectful of both the plant and of life."

CHAPTER 11

A Love Story

My plants have aphids. Again. Or maybe, still. Great masses of them all up and down the stems, all over the leaves. Not just the young plants, but the plants nearly ready for harvest. I'm not going to use chemicals. I don't want to buy more ladybugs, because they're wild-caught, and if I were a ladybug I wouldn't want to be caught, put in a refrigerator, mailed to someone, and put in a hothouse. I'd rather live my life like I'm supposed to, in the wild. And I don't want to buy any *Beauveria bassiana* insect-eating fungus—which I should have bought in the first place and will buy next time—because since I bought the ladybugs they've had several generations of babies, and because I was responsible for their ancestors being removed from the wild, it would be ungrateful for me to now add in a fungus who will eat them from the inside out.

So I figure I'll feed the aphids to the birds.

I take the plants outside.

When I spoke before about birds eating aphids like me eating potato chips, I gave short shrift to predatory insects.

Within five minutes of me taking out the plants, scores of wasps arrive, landing on fan leaves and excitedly feeling/smelling with their antennae. They're not here to eat aphids, but honeydew, which they clearly smelled from a distance.

That's okay. I don't mind feeding wasps.

I go out again a couple of days later and this time see hundreds of tiny wasps of a half-dozen species, anywhere from one thirty-second to half an inch. And hundreds more black smudges on the undersides of leaves. I look at these through a magnifier, and they're wasps the size of the dot over this *i*.

The wasps we hear most about are social wasps, but most species of wasps are solitary and parasitoid. Parasitoids are different than parasites in that parasites don't generally kill their hosts. Parasitoids necessarily do. Parasitoid wasps are exquisitely fascinating, so long as you aren't one their hosts/victims. Then they're terrifying. Most parasitoid wasps have specific hosts, whether those hosts are spiders, caterpillars, cockroaches, or in this case aphids. The wasp finds a host, stings it, then lays an egg in or on it. In some cases, the sting paralyzes the host, who is then dragged to a nest and slowly consumed by the baby wasp. The sting paralyzes rather than kills so the meat will remain fresh. In some cases the sting zombifies the host, so that a spider might spin not a web but instead a cocoon in which the baby wasp will eventually pupate, and a cockroach might become docile and allow itself to be led to the nest where it will be consumed. Since aphids' primary defense is neither to run nor to fight but instead to reproduce as quickly as possible, the wasps just need to insert an egg. The egg grows inside the aphid—in some cases becoming twice as big as the aphid herself—pupates, and then emerges like that scene in *Alien*. As long as I've known about parasitoid wasps, I have prayed that as their victims/hosts are consumed, they're at least in a coma, or dreaming, rather than being fully aware that they're being consumed from the inside out, and there is naught they can do about it.[1]

I'd unintentionally created a feast for tiny wasps who, too, must have smelled the aphids from a distance.

Because it takes ten days or two weeks to go from egg to emerging wasp, I didn't harvest the leaves for a while; I didn't want to juice the wasps and turn this feast into a death trap for generations of wild parasitoid wasps.

I went out a few nights later—just because I love looking at the plants and all the goings on surrounding them—and saw clouds of midges. I pulled out my magnifier and a flashlight and saw little orange grubs crawling along the undersides of leaves. I went inside, asked Ms.

---

[1] Although some caterpillars have been known to eat just the right amount of toxic leaves to kill the wasp larvae while not killing themselves.

Google, and learned of the existence of species of midges who lay eggs in soil, quickly leading to small orange grubs who love to eat—you guessed it—aphids.

Isn't nature magnificent in its complexity: from the existence of 37 million-year-old plants who produce chemicals that somehow combine with our 200 million-year-old endocannabinoid system to the existence of 280 million-year-old insects nearly invisible to the naked eye who want to eat those plants, and who defend against predation by becoming pregnant even before they themselves are born, and who reproduce so prodigiously that despite their infinitesimal size they're important and sometimes sole food sources for other beings; to the existence of predatory insects, 247 million years old, also nearly invisible to the naked eye, who can smell these tiny herbivorous insects from what at least to them must seem miles and miles away?

This book began with me riding in a car, afraid of police, and it ends as it should, with me in love with the marvel that is this plant called *cannabis*—and even more in love with the marvel that is all of life and evolution on this planet, evolution that gave us our endocannabinoid system, that gave all of us—not just humans, but aphids, wasps, and yes, stoned little mousies who eat the buds and fall asleep—this wonderful plant.

About the Authors

DERRICK JENSEN

Derrick Jensen is the author of more than twenty-five books, including *Bright Green Lies, A Language Older Than Words, The Culture of Make Believe,* and *Endgame.* He is also a teacher, activist, and small farmer, and was named the "poet-philosopher of the ecological movement" by Democracy Now! In 2008, he was chosen as one of *Utne Reader's* "50 Visionaries Who Are Changing Your World" and won the Eric Hoffer Award. He is a cofounder of the organization Deep Green Resistance. Jensen has written for the *New York Times Magazine, Audubon Magazine,* and *The Sun,* and was a columnist at *Orion Magazine.* He holds an MFA in creative writing from Eastern Washington University and a BS degree in mineral engineering physics from the Colorado School of Mines, and has taught creative writing at Eastern Washington University and Pelican Bay State Prison. He lives in Northern California on a property frequented by bears.

TONY SILVAGGIO

Tony Silvaggio is an associate professor of Sociology at Humboldt State University and founding faculty member of the Humboldt Institute for Interdisciplinary Marijuana Research. His research focuses on understanding the environmental consequences of cannabis prohibition and the limits of state-level legalization efforts, identifying the ways in which legalization efforts continue to facilitate environmental degradation. One of the first scholars in the United States to sound the alarm about the ecological impacts of industrial cannabis agriculture, he organized the *Earth Day Symposium on Marijuana and the Environment (2013)*, which brought together cannabis cultivators, policymakers, land managers, tribal leaders, law enforcement, and environmentalists to examine the environmental impacts of industrial cannabis agriculture. His most recent work can be found in, *Where There's Smoke: The Environmental Science, Public Policy, and Politics of Marijuana (2018)*. His research has been featured in the *New York Times, The Atlantic, Rolling Stone, Al Jazeera,* and *The Nation.*

CPSIA information can be obtained
at www.ICGtesting.com
Printed in the USA
LVHW011050310322
714806LV00003B/273

9 781954 744554